Bottled and Sold

Bottled and Sold

THE STORY BEHIND
OUR OBSESSION WITH
BOTTLED WATER

~

Peter H. Gleick

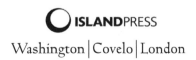

ISLANDPRESS

Washington | Covelo | London

ISLAND PRESS is a trademark of the Center for Resource Economics.

Library of Congress Cataloging-in-Publication Data
Gleick, Peter H.
  Bottled and sold : the story behind our obsession with bottled water /
Peter H. Gleick.
     p. cm.
  Includes bibliographical references and index.
  ISBN-13: 978-1-59726-528-7 (cloth : alk. paper)
  ISBN-10: 1-59726-528-4 (cloth : alk. paper)
  1. Bottled water. I. Title.
  TP659.G54 2010
  663'.61—dc22

                          2009048139

British Cataloguing-in-Publication data available.
Printed on recycled, acid-free paper.⊛

Design by Joyce C. Weston
Manufactured in the United States of America
10 9 8 7 6 5 4 3 2 1

To my closest friend, companion, and love,
Nicki Norman.

∼

Contents

Preface   ix

Chapter 1   The War on Tap Water   1

Chapter 2   Fear of the Tap   15

Chapter 3   Selling Unwholesome Provisions   33

Chapter 4   If It's Called "Arctic Spring," Why Is It from Florida?   51

Chapter 5   The Cachet of Spring Water   63

Chapter 6   The Taste of Water   79

Chapter 7   The Hidden Cost of Convenience   87

Chapter 8   Selling Bottled Water: The Modern Medicine Show   109

Chapter 9   Drinking Bottled Water: Sin or Salvation?   131

Chapter 10   Revolt: The Growing Campaign Against Bottled Water   143

Chapter 11   Green Water? The Effort to Produce Ethical Bottled Water   163

Chapter 12   The Future of Water   171

Acknowledgments   181

Notes   183

Index   203

A Thousand Bottles a Second

THINK ABOUT WHERE you are right now. How far away is the nearest faucet with safe water? Probably not very far. Yet every second of every day in the United States, a thousand people buy and open up a plastic bottle of commercially produced water, and every second of every day in the United States, a thousand plastic bottles are thrown away. Eighty-five million bottles a day. More than thirty billion bottles a year at a cost to consumers of tens of billions of dollars. And for every bottle consumed in the U.S., another four are consumed around the world.

Why do we buy bottled water? Where does it come from? What's really in the bottles we buy? Is it as safe as tap water, or even safer, as we are often told? What about the plastic? Where do those bottles go when we throw them out? What are the environmental and social consequences of bottled water use for the planet? The beverage industry tells us that bottled water is just a simple commodity like any other food product—a safe, well-regulated alternative to tap water. The environmental community tells us bottled water is a corporate plot to privatize a precious public resource and that it's even less safe than our tap water. What is the truth?

I decided to write this book in part to gain a better understanding of what the explosive growth of the bottled water industry really means for us and for the future of drinking water. In the course of writing it, I've interviewed people who have made a business out of bottling and selling water, met with passionate environmental activists vociferously opposed to bottled water, visited the factories where petroleum and raw water are turned into neat little containers of commercial product, and looked out over acres of plastic waste and the landfills where that waste will end up lying intact for centuries. I believe that bottled water is a symptom of a larger set of issues: the long-term decay of our public water systems, inequitable access to safe water around the world, our susceptibility to advertising and marketing, and a society trained from birth to buy, consume, and throw away. I believe that bottled water can only be understood within the broader context of these phenomena.

The globe is in the midst of a major transition to what I call the Third Water Age—a transition to a truly sustainable system of managing and using our most precious resource. The First Age began when humans emerged as thinking beings and depended on the vagaries of the natural hydrologic cycle to take what water was needed and to get rid of wastes. The transition to the Second Water Age began when humanity started to outgrow the limits of local water resources and to intentionally manipulate the hydrologic cycle, building the earliest dams, aqueducts, irrigation canals, and wastewater systems, and putting in place the first laws and social structures for managing water. The Second Water Age reached full flower in the nineteenth and twentieth centuries when societies began to master the complex chemical, engineering, biological, and institutional tools that characterize our modern water systems. The Second Age brought us enormous benefits but has ultimately proven inadequate to the growing need. Billions of people still lack safe water and sanitation. Aquatic ecosystems continue to be devastated by our use, diversion, and contamination of fresh water. Conflicts over shared water resources are growing. Climate changes are already altering the planet's fundamental hydrological conditions.

The growing use of bottled water is further evidence that the old ways of managing our limited water resources are on the wrong side of history and that a new way of thinking is needed. We are now, I believe, in the midst of another transition, to a Third Water Age. My fear is that this Third Age could consist of the complete abandonment of our efforts to provide safe public tap water for all in favor of privately produced and sold bottled water. My hope is that the Third Age will instead follow a "soft path" for water—a comprehensive approach to sustainable water management and use, requiring equitable access to water, proper application and use of economics, comprehensive protection of aquatic ecosystems, incentives for efficient water use, new sources of supply, smart use of innovative technology, improved water quality and delivery reliability, strong public participation in decision-making, and more. In my vision of Third Age, access to affordable safe tap water would be universal and bottled water use would become unnecessary. Government regulatory agencies would successfully protect the public from water contamination, false advertising, misleading marketing, and blatant hucksterism. Public access to drinking water would be easy, and selling bottled water would be difficult. And while bottled water will always be an option for those that want it, in this positive vision of the future bottled water companies would have to incorporate the true economic and environmental costs of the production and disposal of plastic bottles, as well as the extraction and use of sensitive groundwater, into the price of their product, further drying up bottled water sales. But this future vision is not today's reality: none of these things are true now, and so we buy bottled water. Lots of it.

The story of bottled water is a story with big numbers: billions of gallons or liters sold; billions of bottles produced, used, and thrown away; tens or hundreds of billions of dollars in sales; billions of tons of carbon dioxide and other pollutants produced. But it is also a story about a billion people worldwide without access to safe and affordable drinking water, and billions of illnesses and millions of deaths every year—mostly among small children—from preventable water-related diseases.

People usually say they buy bottled water for four major reasons: fear of their tap water, convenience, taste, and style. The news is filled with stories about water contamination and so we start to fear that our tap water is polluted by things we cannot see or smell. We seek the convenience of little portable packages of water that are available wherever and whenever we want them because we can no longer find a clean, working water fountain. Sometimes we really don't like how our tap water tastes. And we're misled by intensive advertising into believing that this or that brand of commercial water will make us healthier, skinnier, or more popular.

So we've turned to the bottle, convinced that paying a thousand times more for individually packaged plastic throwaway containers of water than for readily available tap water is an act of rationality rather than economic, environmental, and social blindness. Whether or not we are right is a question to which I'll return in many ways throughout this book, but we should not lose sight of the fact that while we turn away from the tap, the poorest people in the poorest countries of the world, who have neither safe tap water nor money to buy bottled water, drink whatever is available, get sick, and often die. This dichotomy leads to a strange reality: Suburban shoppers in America lug cases of plastic water bottles from the grocery store back to homes supplied with unlimited piped potable water in a sad and unintentional parody of the labor of girls and women in Africa, who spend countless backbreaking hours carrying containers of filthy water from distant contaminated sources to homes with no water at all.

I confess to conflicting and ambiguous feelings about bottled water. On rare occasions I will buy and consume bottled water. The flaws of the entire bottled water industry are so clear and obvious that they deserve attention and redress, and I describe them in this book. Yet bottled water is neither the cause of, nor the solution to, our larger water problems. If bottled water were to magically disappear tomorrow or somehow be banned from our stores, our global water problems and the need to pursue the soft path would still remain. The bottled water companies argue that the problems and concerns that cause people to buy bottled water are not the fault of the industry; rather, they say the industry is responding to a demand that results from flaws in our water system that they did not cause and are not in a position to fix. This argument cannot be dismissed lightly. There are many places on this planet where tap water is unsafe or unavailable because of the failure of governments to meet the basic needs of their people.

But the bottled water companies cannot be held completely blameless—some of them are no better than old-time snake-oil salesmen peddling magic potions or worthless health elixirs. At times, they have subtly and even openly worked to disparage tap water and to sow fear of unseen contamination in order to boost their own sales. They have pressed hard to prevent effective and comprehensive plastic recycling programs. And they have used the classic advertising and marketing tools of sex, fear, style, and image to drive people toward their product and away from the tap.

What's really at stake? In the end, the arguments for and against bottled water are more than simply environmental or economic. The arguments have deeper psychological underpinnings, philosophical and ideological implications, and social subtexts about public rights versus private goods, the human right to water, free markets, the appropriate role of governments, and conflicting visions of the future. Contrasting forces are also at work, including the antiglobalization movement, the growing effort to be "green," and the newly awakened concern about climate change and its root cause—our style and extent of energy use. These are all part of the forces that are driving the new transition to the Third Water Age.

It is possible that we will look back in a few decades at a short-lived bottled water craze and wonder what we were thinking. But if we don't address our growing water crisis, we could just as easily look back wistfully at the era of safe, cheap, and reliable tap water as a golden age when, for a little while, we could just turn on our faucets and drink to our hearts' content.

Peter Gleick
Berkeley, California

CHAPTER 1

The War on Tap Water

Tap water is poison.
— A flyer touting the stock of a Texas
bottled water company.

When we're done, tap water will be relegated to showers and
washing dishes.
— Susan Wellington, president of the Quaker Oats
Company's United States beverage division.

SEPTEMBER 15, 2007, was a big day for the alumni, family, and
fans of the University of Central Florida and the UCF Knights football team. After years of waiting and hoping, the University of Central Florida had finally built their own football stadium—the new
Bright House Networks arena. Under clear skies, and with temperatures nearing 100 degrees, a sell-out crowd of 45,622 was on hand to
watch the first-ever real UCF home game against the Texas Long-
horns, a national powerhouse. "I never thought we'd see this, but we
sure are proud to have a stadium on campus," said UCF alumnus
and Knight fan Tim Ball as he and his family tailgated in the parking
lot before the game. And in an exciting, three-hour back-and-forth
contest, the UCF Knights almost pulled off an upset before losing in
the final minutes 35 to 32.

Knight supporters were thrilled and left thirsting for more—
literally. Fans found out the hard way that their new $54-million sta-
dium had been built without a single drinking water fountain. And

for "security" reasons, no one could bring water into the stadium. The only water available for overheated fans was $3 bottled water from the concessionaires or water from the bathroom taps, and long before the end of the game, the concessionaires had run out of bottled water. Eighteen people were taken to local hospitals and sixty more were treated by campus medical personnel for heat-related illnesses. The 2004 Florida building code, in effect in 2005 when the UCF Board of Trustees approved the stadium design, mandated that stadiums and other public arenas have a water fountain for every 1,000 seats, or half that number if "bottled water dispensers" are available.[1] Under these requirements, the arena should have been built with at least twenty water fountains. Furthermore, a spokesman for the International Code Council in Washington, which developed Florida's building code, said, "Selling bottled water out of a concession stand is not what the code meant."

The initial reaction from the University was swift and remarkably unapologetic: UCF spokesman Grant Heston appeared on the local TV news to argue that the codes in place when the stadium was designed didn't require fountains. A few days after the game, as news of the hospitalizations was reverberating, University President John Hitt said, "We will look at adding the water fountains, but I have to say to you I don't think that's the answer to this problem. We could have had 50 water fountains and still had a problem on Saturday."[2] Al Harms, UCF's vice president for strategic planning and the coordinator for the operations of the stadium, told the Orlando Sentinel, "We won't make a snap decision" about installing fountains in the new stadium. Harms did promise that they would triple the amount of bottled water available for sale, and give away one free bottle per person at the next game.[3] Harms also said, apparently without a trace of sarcasm, "It's our way of saying we're sorry."

For some UCF students, this wasn't enough. One of them, Nathaniel Dorn, mobilized in twenty-first-century fashion. He created a Facebook group, Knights for Free Water, which quickly attracted nearly 700 members. He and several other students showed up at a packed school hearing, talked to local TV and print media, and ridiculed the school's offer of a free bottle of water. Under this glare of attention the University did an abrupt about-face and announced that ten fountains would be installed by the next game and fifty would be installed permanently.

All of a sudden public water fountains have vanished and bottled water is everywhere: in every convenience store, beverage cooler, and vending machine. In student backpacks, airplane beverage carts, and all of my hotel rooms. At every conference and meeting I go to. On restaurant menus and school lunch counters. In early 2007, as I waited for a meeting in Silicon Valley, I watched a steady stream of young employees pass by on their way to or from buildings on the Google campus. Nearly all were carrying two items: a laptop and a throw-away plastic bottle of water. When I entered the lobby and checked in at reception, I was told to help myself to something to drink from an open cooler containing fruit juices and rows of commercial bottled water. As I walked to my meeting, I passed cases of bottled water being unloaded near the cafeteria.

Water fountains used to be everywhere, but they have slowly disappeared as public water is increasingly pushed out in favor of private control and profit. Water fountains have become an anachronism, or even a liability, a symbol of the days when homes didn't have taps and bottled water wasn't available from every convenience store and corner concession stand. In our health-conscious society, we're afraid that public fountains, and our tap water in general, are sources of contamination and contagion. It used to be the exact opposite—in the 1800s, when our cities lacked widespread access to safe water, there were major movements to build free public water fountains throughout America and Europe.

In London in the mid-1800s, water was beginning to be piped directly into the homes of the city's wealthier inhabitants. The poor, however, relied on private water vendors and neighborhood wells that were often broken or tainted by contamination and disease, like the famous Broad Street pump that spread cholera throughout its neighborhood. At the time of London's Great Exhibition in 1851, conceived to showcase the triumphs of British technology, science, and innovation, *Punch Magazine* wrote: "Whoever can produce in London a glass of water fit to drink will contribute the best and most universally useful article in the whole exhibition."[4] Just three years after the Exhibition, thousands of Londoners would die in the third massive cholera outbreak to hit the city since 1800.

By the middle of the twentieth century, spectacular efforts to improve water-quality treatment and major investments in modern drinking-water systems had almost completely eliminated the risks of unsafe water. Those of us who have the good fortune to live in the industrialized world now take safe drinking water entirely for granted. We turn on a faucet and out comes safe, often free fresh water. Notwithstanding the UCF stadium fiasco, we're rarely more than a few feet from potable water no matter where we are. But those efforts and investments are in danger of being wasted, and the public benefit of safe tap water lost, in favor of private gain in the form of little plastic water bottles.

The growth of the bottled water industry is a story about twenty-first-century controversies and contradictions: poverty versus glitterati; perception versus reality; private gain versus public loss. Today people visit luxury water "bars" stocked with bottles of water shipped in from every corner of the world. Water "sommeliers" at fancy restaurants push premium bottled water to satisfy demand and boost profits. Airport travelers have no choice but to buy bottled water at exorbitant prices because their own personal water is considered a security risk. Celebrities tout their current favorite brands of bottled water to fans. People with too much money and too little sense pay $50 or more for plain water in a fancy glass bottle covered in fake gems, or for "premium" water supposedly bottled in some exotic place or treated with some magical process.

In its modern form, bottled water is a new phenomenon, growing from a niche mineral-water product with a few wealthy customers to a global commodity found almost everywhere. The recent expansion of bottled water sales has been extraordinary. In the late 1970s, around 350 million gallons of bottled water were sold in the United States—almost entirely sparkling mineral water and large bottles to supply office water coolers—or little more than a gallon and a half per person per year. As the figure below shows, between 1976 and 2008, sales of bottled water in the United States doubled, doubled again, doubled again, and then doubled *again*. In 2008, nearly 9 *billion* gallons (over 34 billion liters) of bottled water were packaged and sold in the United States and five times this amount was sold around the world, feeding a global business of water providers, bottlers, truckers, and retailers at a cost to consumers of over a hundred billion dollars.

Americans now drink more bottled water than milk or beer—in fact, the average American is now drinking around 30 gallons, or 115

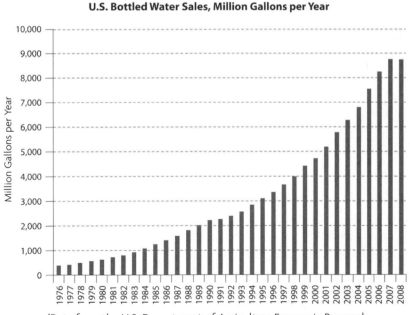

U.S. Bottled Water Sales, Million Gallons per Year

(Data from the U.S. Department of Agriculture Economic Research Service and the Beverage Marketing Corporation.)

liters, of bottled water each year, most of it from single-serving plastic containers. Bottled water has become so ubiquitous that it's hard to remember that it hasn't always been here. As I write this sentence I'm sitting in the café in the basement of the capitol building in Sacramento, California, and all I have to do is lift my eyes from my computer screen—right in front of me are vending machines selling both Dasani and Aquafina. Yet, like UCF football fans, I can't tell you where the nearest water fountain is.

Millions of Americans still drink tap water at home and in restaurants. But there is a war on for the hearts, minds, and pocketbooks of tap water drinkers, a huge market that water bottlers cannot afford to ignore. The war on the tap is an undeclared war, for the most part, but in recent years, more and more subtle (and not so subtle) campaigns that play up the supposed health risks of tap water, or the supposed health advantages of bottled water, have been launched by private water bottlers.

How do you convince consumers to buy something that is essentially the same as a far cheaper and more easily accessible alternative? You promote perceived advantages of your product, and you emphasize the flaws in your competitor's product. For water bottlers this means selling safety, style, and convenience, and playing on consumer's fears. Fear is an effective tool. Especially fear of sickness and of invisible contamination. If we can be made to fear our tap water, the market for bottled water skyrockets.

I guess I shouldn't have been surprised, therefore, when I opened my mailbox and found a flyer with a cover image of a goldfish swimming in a glass of drinking water. "There is something in this glass you do not want to drink. And it's not the fish," shouted the bold and colorful text in the mailer, offering me home delivery of bottles of Calistoga Mountain Spring Water. "How can you be sure your water is safe? Take a closer look at the water in our glass. Can you tell if it's pure? Unfortunately, you can't." And the solution offered? The "Path to Purity" lies with bottles of water, delivered to your door by truck, under a monthly contract.

"Tap water is poison!" declares another flyer my neighbor Roy received in the mail in early 2007 touting the stock of Royal Spring Water Inc., a Texas bottled water company. "Americans no longer trust their tap water. . . . Clearly, people are more worried than ever about what comes out of their taps." Roy, a thoughtful guy, told me he was actually more worried about what came out of his mailbox than his tap. The website of another bottler says, "Tap water can be inconsistent. . . . The U.S. Environmental Protection Agency has reported that hundreds of tap water sources have failed to meet minimum standards."5

These attacks could be dismissed as the inappropriate actions of a few small players, except that some of the world's biggest bottlers have also targeted tap water. In 2000, shortly before he was made chairman of PepsiCo's North American Beverage and Food division, Robert S. Morrison publicly declared, "The biggest enemy is tap water. . . . We're not against water—it just has its place. We think it's good for irrigation and cooking."6 That same year, Susan Wellington, president of the Quaker Oats Company's United States beverage division, candidly told industry analysts, "When we're done, tap water will be relegated to showers and washing dishes."7 "We need to change the way we sell water," said industry analyst Kathleen Ransome at the 2006 International Bottled Water Association annual convention in Las Vegas. "At what point will consumers turn to the tap?"8

Subtler advertising approaches also play on our fears. PepsiCo hired actress Lisa Kudrow to promote Aquafina with the phrase "So pure, we promise nothing" in a campaign Brandweek magazine jokingly called the "Nothing" campaign.9 Kinley in India offers "Trust in every drop," while another Indian bottler, Bisleri, advertises "Bisleri. Play safe."

Officially, the large bottled water industry associations advise their members to refrain from attacks on tap water. Some bottled water companies have signed up to the International Bottled Water Association's voluntary code of advertising, "which encourages members not to disparage tap water."[10] Alas, as Captain Barbossa notes in the popular movie *Pirates of the Caribbean*, "the code is more what you'd call 'guidelines' than actual rules," and even the bottled water associations cannot resist making critical comments about tap water. "The difference between bottled water and tap water is that bottled water's quality is consistent," said Stephen Kay, IBWA spokesman in May 2001, implying, of course, that tap water quality isn't and thus worse.[11] In 2002, Kay said, "Some people in their municipal markets have the luxury of good water. Others do not."[12] Similarly, the website of the Australasian Bottled Water Association pokes barbs at tap water, saying, "Some people also wish to avoid certain chemicals used in the treatment of public water supplies, such as chlorine and fluoride, and are therefore turning to the chemical-free alternative."[13]

In the fall of 2007 I attended the IBWA annual convention in Las Vegas. Las Vegas is a pretty incongruous place to hold a bottled water convention. Planted in the heart of one of the driest regions in the United States, it has very limited access to water. Yet the IBWA's major social event is a golf tournament played on water-intensive grass that consumes precious, limited water. The bottled water convention itself is a cross between a pep rally, a political campaign meeting, and a how-to seminar for individuals hoping to cash in on the bottled water craze. I wandered from session to session, from discussions of marketing strategies to closed-door meetings on how to deal with new regulatory efforts by federal agencies. I listened to talks on how to counter the efforts of anti–bottled water activists and watched demonstrations of the latest machines for bottling water. The culmination of the convention was the keynote presentation of Fred Smith, president of the Competitive Enterprise Institute, which promotes a libertarian, free-market agenda.[14] Smith extolled the virtues of a world where business entrepreneurs could make money selling water in bottles. The problem, Smith told me afterward, without a hint of irony, was that water "suffers most from being treated as a common property resource." Smith believes that "water policy could benefit greatly from exploring the strategies that have been used to produce oil."[15]

It is this belief that water is fundamentally no different than oil or any other private commodity that lies at the heart of the controversy over selling water. A few months after the IBWA convention, Smith's Competitive Enterprise Institute launched a special project called "Enjoy Bottled Water" in which they criticize the safety of tap water, ridicule opponents of bottled water, and promote the industry's merits. "Bottled water is substantially different from tap water," the CEI website declares. "When compared to bottled water, risks appear to be somewhat higher for tap water. . . . Available data indicates that bottled water has a better safety record." The CEI is so ideologically anti-regulation that the site says, "The fact that anyone would want to ban or regulate a healthy and safe option like bottled water is really absurd."[16] It may come as no surprise to note that Coca-Cola, maker of Dasani bottled water, was the largest single supporter of CEI's annual fundraising dinner in 2008.[17]

The campaign against municipal tap water has been more than just words. In 2001, documents found on a Coca-Cola company website revealed that it had a formal program to actively discourage restaurant customers from drinking tap water. Working with the Olive Garden restaurant chain, Coca-Cola developed a six-step program to help the restaurant reduce what they call "tap water incidence"—the unprofitable problem of customers drinking tap water rather than ordering revenue-producing beverages. "Some 20 percent of consumers drink tap water exclusively in Casual Dining restaurants," the program lamented. "This trend significantly cuts into retailer profits. . . . Research was conducted to better understand why tap water consumption is so prevalent and why consumers are making this beverage choice. . . . This research provides the valuable insight and understanding needed to convert water drinkers to profit-producing beverages."[18]

These documents, very quickly pulled from official websites when the media picked up the story, had already been downloaded and reposted elsewhere. "This is awesome," commented one reader. "It's what corporations say to each other behind customers' backs, only it happens to be on the Web where mortals can see it."[19]

It isn't just bottled water companies that have tap water in their sights. Full-service restaurants have recognized the profit-generating potential of bottled water. Servers in restaurants operated by the Omni Hotels and Resorts, for example, are trained to describe "the characteristics of the waters being offered and are also trained to approach the table with chilled bottles of water. They offer it to the guest as an option to tap water," according to Fernando Salazar, corporate director of the food and beverage division in 2006. "It's just part of the server's presentation to offer bottled water first before offering tap water," says Salazar. "Those restaurants that are not yet doing this are missing an opportunity to increase profits."[20]

Brita, a subsidiary of the Clorox Company that sells home water filters, has also been particularly aggressive in maligning tap water, which is their direct competitor in the home market. One of Brita's advertising campaigns claimed that a Brita filter "turns tap water into drinking water." Other Brita ads say, "We'd like to clear up a few things about tap water." "Tap water becomes wonderful water." "Too often, impurities are finding their way into the water. While you may not be able to see them, you don't want them."[21] One of Brita's television ads aired in the United States and Canada took a particularly graphic approach, with the camera focused on a glass of water in a kitchen. Viewers watch the glass drain and then refill to the background sound of a flushing toilet. Superimposed on the image were the words "Tap and toilet water come from the same source," and the voice-over at the end of the commercial asked viewers: "Don't you deserve better?" In the magazine version, the advertising copy read, "You deserve better than the water you mop with."[22]

These efforts sparked the ire of both the American Water Works Association, which represents municipal water agencies, and its Canadian counterpart. The Associations publicly objected to Brita's "unsavory tactics" and called on Brita to cancel the commercials.

Advertising Standards Canada, which regulates advertising, received eleven formal complaints and after reviewing the ads ruled that they "conveyed an inaccurate representation of a product/service/ commercial activity; omitted relevant information; unfairly demeaned, disparaged, and discredited another product/service/commercial activity (i.e., municipally supplied water); and misled consumers by playing upon their fears of the safety of drinking water."[23]

Looking at the massive growth in bottled water consumption, it is apparent that the bottled water companies have been winning the war against tap water. And in one of their latest campaign tactics, the bottled water industry is now arguing in debates, Congressional testimony, advertising, and media campaigns that the growth of bottled water sales doesn't come at the expense of tap water, but rather other commercial beverages. In 2003, Stephen Kay, spokesman for the International Bottled Water Association, told *E—The Environmental Magazine* that "bottled water's competition is soft drinks, not tap water."[24] In 2006, he told the *Chicago Tribune's* "Morning Call" column that "bottled water's competition is not your faucet but the soft drinks, juices, sport drinks, and teas that people buy while they're on the go."[25]

The industry continues to push this argument. In August 2007, they bought full-page ads in the *New York Times* and other papers. "Whether it comes from a faucet or a bottle, drinking water is an easy step people can take to lead a healthier lifestyle. So, as far as we're concerned, the drink in everyone's purse, backpack, and lunch box should be water." In December 2007, in testimony to the U.S. Congress, the IBWA President, Joe Doss, said, "Consumers also choose bottled water over other beverages because it does not contain calories, caffeine, sugar, artificial flavors or colors, alcohol and other ingredients."[26] Bottled water consumption is good, the industry argues, because the growth of bottled water sales has come not at the expense of tap water, but of other beverages.

This is an intriguing and potentially powerful argument, except that it is false. After hearing the industry repeat this claim over and

over, I went and looked up the actual numbers. Are we really drinking bottled water instead of soft drinks and other consumer beverages, as the industry argues, or are we actually drinking less tap
water? The U.S. Department of Commerce collects and publishes
excellent data on beverage consumption. Contrary to what the bottled water industry argues, the numbers show that we are buying
more bottled water *and* carbonated soft drinks, and drinking less of
everything else, including milk, coffee, tea, fruit juices, beer, wine,
hard alcohol, and especially tap water.

The graph below clearly shows the growth in consumption of
both soft drinks and bottled water at the expense of everything else
we drink. Indeed, between 1980 and 2006, data on beverage consumption reveals that on average, each of us is actually drinking
around 36 gallons per year *less* tap water now. With what have we
replaced this water? Soda and bottled water. Over this same period of
time, our consumption of carbonated soft drinks has grown by 17

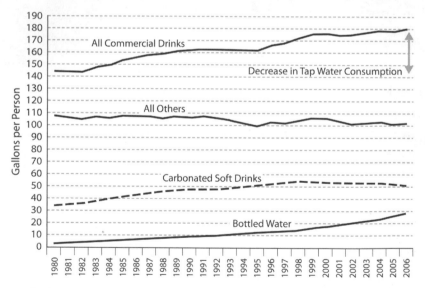

Commercial Beverage Sales in the U.S. in Gallons per Person per Year

The increase in beverage sales has led to a decrease in tap water consumption.
(Data from the U.S. Department of Agriculture Economic Research Service.)

gallons per person per year, our consumption of bottled water has grown by 25 gallons per person per year, and our purchases of all other beverages, including milk, juices, beer, tea, coffee, and hard liquor have dropped by 6 gallons per year.

The beverage companies are winning the war on tap water. As long as people can be made to fear tap water, they will seek out alternatives they think offer more safety. But we have to ask: is bottled water actually any safer? What do we know about what's actually in our tap water—or in the bottles of water we buy? And how safe is it to drink?

The label says Fiji because it's not bottled in Cleveland.

Why would anyone travel halfway around the world for a drink of water? More importantly, why would anyone go through all that trouble to bring it back? After all, it's just water. Or is it?

FIJI Water is only found in one of the most remote places on the planet, thousands of miles from the nearest industrialized continent, at the very edge of a primitive rainforest.

Our water begins as rain, purified by equatorial trade winds after traveling thousands of miles across the Pacific Ocean. Once it arrives in Fiji, it filters through volcanic rock over hundreds of years. During this process, FIJI Water collects life-essential minerals, like silica, and finally gathers in a natural artesian aquifer, where it is preserved and protected from external elements.

Bottled at the source, natural artesian pressure forces the water through a hermetically sealed delivery system free of human contact.

In Fiji, we believe bottled water should be as rare and uncompromised as its source. That's why FIJI Water will always be created by, bottled in, and shipped to you from the islands of Fiji.

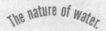

The nature of water.

CHAPTER 2

Fear of the Tap

Water, water, every where
Nor any drop to drink.
— Samuel Taylor Coleridge, *The Rime of the
Ancient Mariner*

IN JULY 2006 the City of Cleveland's public utilities director Julius Ciaccia opened his e-mail to find a message from a colleague asking him if he had seen the full page Fiji Water advertisement running in the most current issue of *Esquire* and other national magazines. Fiji Water sells spring water actually produced in and shipped from the remote South Pacific island nation of Fiji. The ad showed a picture of the trademark square Fiji water bottle, with the headline: "The label says Fiji because it's not bottled in Cleveland."

Poor Cleveland. The city was founded in the early 1800s on the shores of Lake Erie, one of the largest bodies of fresh water on the planet, but it has never had an easy time with water supply. Cleveland's first water-delivery system consisted of Benhu Johnson, a one-legged veteran of the War of 1812, two barrels, and a wagon pulled by a pony. Johnson would deliver a gallon of Lake Erie water to anyone willing to pay 2 cents. The city rapidly outgrew Benhu and his pony, and by the beginning of the Civil War, Cleveland was operating a sophisticated water system of pumps, reservoirs, and distribution pipelines delivering 38,000 gallons a day.

By the mid-1960s, however, untreated municipal and industrial wastes from U.S. and Canadian cities had turned Lake Erie into a dead zone, and on June 22, 1969, Americans turned on the national news to see the Cuyahoga River running through Cleveland on fire. This iconic image made Cleveland the butt of jokes for decades and, incidentally, led to a great Randy Newman song, "Burn on," with the following lyrics:

> Cleveland, even now I can remember
> 'Cause the Cuyahoga River
> Goes smokin' through my dreams
>
> Burn on, big river, burn on
> Burn on, big river, burn on
> Now the Lord can make you tumble
> And the Lord can make you turn
> And the Lord can make you overflow
> But the Lord can't make you burn.[1]

This incident, however, also led to the federal Clean Water Act of 1972, the Great Lakes Water Quality Agreement, and the creation of the U.S. Environmental Protection Agency (EPA). Today, Lake Erie is far cleaner than it's been in years, and Cleveland's water system provides 90 billion gallons of high-quality potable water to customers every year. Two cents today will pay for nearly 30 gallons of water of a far higher quality than Benhu Johnson and his pony were able to deliver.

It should be no surprise then to find out that Ciaccia, responsible for managing Cleveland's water system, was not amused by the Fiji ad. After seeing it, Ciaccia ordered the city water-quality department to test Fiji Water. The results? While both Fiji Water and Cleveland's tap water met all federal standards, the lab tests reportedly indicated that Fiji Water contained volatile plastic compounds, 40 times more bacteria than are found in well-run municipal water systems, and most noticeably, over six micrograms per liter of arsenic. Cleveland tap water had no measurable arsenic. And while six micrograms per liter is within U.S. regulatory limits, Cleveland was offered a priceless opportunity to strike back at Fiji Water. The media picked up the story, and soon Fiji Water had more publicity than it wanted, and the wrong kind. "Don't tread on Cleveland water," said the local *Cleveland Plain-Dealer.* "Cleveland gets testy over bottled water," wrote the *Pittsburgh Post-Gazette.* "Cleveland takes offense at Fiji Water ad," echoed the *Washington Post.* "Before you take a cheap shot at somebody, know what you're talking about," said Cleveland water commissioner J. Christopher Nielson. Edward Cochran, Fiji Water president, weakly tried to defend the company, saying, "It is only a joke. We had to pick some town," days before pulling the ad. In December 2006 the Fiji Water advertisement was voted number 20 on CNN's list of the 101 Dumbest Moments in Business in 2006.[2]

What Fiji and other bottlers understand is that people can be made to fear the quality of the water that comes out of their taps. We don't know where it comes from. We don't know what's done to purify it. And we're distrustful of the governments or corporations that have the responsibility to clean, protect, and deliver it. As a result, many people seek out alternatives, and the bottled water industry is happy to take advantage of this distrust. They subtly and blatantly play on our fears to boost sales through advertising and marketing, and through campaigns to move consumers from tap water to the bottle. The irony is that, behind the scenes, most local water systems do a remarkable job of ensuring a clean water supply, most of the time.

I never saw bottled water when I was a child. My mother never brought home water from the grocery store—and what a bizarre event that would have been. We drank milk or apple juice or New York City tap water. My friends, family, and acquaintances all drank tap water without a second thought. I drank from the faucet, public school drinking fountains, Central Park bubbling fountains in the playgrounds, even an occasional fire hydrant opened up on a hot summer day. New Yorkers bragged about their tap water, and with good reason: the city has one of the purest water supplies of any major metropolitan area.

The public water fountain has a long and noble history. Ancient Greek cities were known for their spectacular public fountains fed by springs and dedicated to gods or heroes. Pausanias, a second-century Greek writer known for his detailed descriptions of ancient Greece, wrote that no place deserves the name of "city" if it lacks such a fountain. Other ancient Greek writers described celebrated fountains at Megara, the Corinthian cities of Peirene and Lerna, and elsewhere.3 Early Rome depended on sophisticated aqueducts to bring water from distant springs to its fountains, public baths, and private villas. According to Frontinus, the *curator aquarum* ("keeper of the aqueducts") in Rome in the first century A.D., Rome had nine aqueducts that fed 39 monumental fountains and 591 public basins. Fountains and public baths in the ancient hill fortress of the Alhambra in Granada, Spain, were fed by *acequias* that still function today.

By the middle of the nineteenth century, however, most of the big cities in Europe lacked decent water-delivery infrastructure to serve exploding populations. Even in Rome, the aqueducts and fountains had long fallen into disrepair, and in London, most of the population relied on contaminated wells or water drawn from the filthy Thames. In 1859, however, a new radical water movement was launched in London by a small group of citizens. Spurred on by the growing control of city water by private water companies and by the lack of other public options, the new Metropolitan Free Drinking Fountain Association chose a simple, yet effective tool: the public water fountain. The mission of the Metropolitan Free Drinking Fountain Association was to build fountains throughout the city "so constructed as to ensure by filters, or other suitable means, the perfect purity and coldness of the water."4 The first Association fountain was built at Saint Sepulchre's church and opened on April 21, 1859. Within a short time, the fountain was being used by 7,000 people a day. This success didn't go unnoticed: by 1872 London had 300 public water fountains and by 1879 nearly 800. Charles Dickens Jr., the son of the famous author, noted in his *Dictionary of London*:

> Until the last few years London was ill-provided with public drinking fountains and cattle troughs. This matter is now well looked after by the Metropolitan Drinking Fountain and Cattle Trough Association, which has erected and is now maintaining nearly 800 fountains and troughs, at which an enormous quantity of water is consumed daily. It is estimated that 300,000 people take advantage of the fountains on a summer's day, and a single trough has supplied the wants of 1,800 horses in one period of 24 hours.[5]

Across the English Channel, in the late 1880s Parisians were getting their own public fountains, ironically contributed by another Englishman, Sir Richard Wallace. Paris, like Rome, has been served over the centuries with potable water from distant sources, including Roman aqueducts and the Canal de l'Ourcq, built during Napoleon's time to bring spring water from 150 kilometers away, as well as local rivers and groundwater aquifers. During the bloody Franco-Prussian war of 1870–71, the city underwent a long siege that destroyed most of Paris's water systems. The poorer populations were unable to pay private vendors for adequate safe water, and water-related diseases started to reappear. Sir Richard Wallace, an eccentric philanthropist who had adopted France as his home, remained in Paris during the siege. When the fighting ended, he devoted substantial parts of his wealth to help rebuild Paris, founding a hospital and funding what became his most visible legacy, "the Wallace Fountains." Wallace worked with sculptor Charles-Auguste Lebourg to design several types of water fountains, and he then paid for their production and installation throughout the city. Many of the green cast-iron foundations remain functional today, providing free potable water to all.

Nineteenth-century American cities also struggled to provide safe water to the public, and water fountains were often provided by prominent citizens and philanthropists. In the 1870s in Detroit, Michigan, Congressman Moses Field petitioned the Detroit Common Council to build public drinking fountains throughout the city. In June of 1871, seven fountains were installed throughout the downtown area and the immediate demand was so great that nine more fountains were ordered the following month. According to records from the city's Board of Public Works, Detroit spent $255.24 that year on fountains. In 1887, an ornate fountain was built in the name of the late John J. Bagley, former governor, police chief, and tobacco magnate. The local newspapers described it as "by far the most elegant of any in the city . . . and cost upwards of $5,000."[6] In August 1881 the circus showman P. T. Barnum donated a public drinking water fountain to his hometown of Bethel, Connecticut, and thousands of townspeople turned out to celebrate.[7] In the early 1900s, when Portland, Oregon, was a lumber town with local saloons and rowdy lumberjacks, a local timber baron, Simon Benson, paid for the installation of twenty public water fountains for his drunken employees, who claimed to have no non-alcoholic alternatives. These ornate, bowl-shaped bronze fountains were designed by A. E. Doyle, a local architect, and the fountains were promptly dubbed "Benson Bubblers." By 1917 the city had installed additional fountains throughout the downtown area.

New York City in the mid-1800s was still a young city compared to its European counterparts, and still inventing its character and form. Like London, New York underwent severe trials and tribulations before a safe water system was put in place. One of New York's most brilliant decisions was to ask designers Frederick Law Olmsted and Calvert Vaux to create what would become the green heart of Manhattan—Central Park. From the very beginning, their plans included ornamental drinking fountains to provide free, safe water in every corner of the park. In May 1886 a public water fountain was unveiled in the city with the inscription "I will give unto him that is athirst of the fountain of the water of life freely," quoting Revelations 21:6.

I grew up in New York, just a couple of blocks from Central Park; in many ways I grew up inside the park and I remember these fountains. My father and I spent hours birding there, wandering from one quiet oasis to another, finding the avian rarities that landed in the park during spring and fall migrations. We knew where all of the water fountains were, often navigating our way from fountain to fountain on days when the rest of the city sweltered. And as a young child in a New York City public school, I ducked and covered my way through the Cuban Missile Crisis in the halls by the white ceramic drinking fountains built into the walls themselves. Our formal pleas to our elementary school teachers of "May I get a drink of water" were certainly as common as "May I go to the bathroom."

But the history of water-related diseases has always left water fountains suspect, despite our efforts to provide clean water. Before cities built municipal water systems to purify tap water and collect and treat wastewater, diseases like dysentery, typhoid, and cholera were rampant, and people avoided drinking just plain water. When the Pilgrims arrived in the New World, their search for a suitable place to settle was cut short, some historians argue, by a crisis brought on by a shortage of their principal drink, beer. A journal entry made on December 19, 1620, by William Bradford, later to be governor of the Plymouth Plantation, notes, "We could not now take time for further search or consideration, our victuals being much spent, especially our beer."[8] No beer? Why was this such a crisis? Because the Pilgrims didn't trust the water and they needed to stop in order to brew an alternative.

Before the medical world gave us the tools to test water and identify contaminants, and before the industrial revolution gave us the tools to purify water, centuries of experience had taught Europeans to avoid it entirely. In the middle of the 1800s, sources of water were the same places we dumped our wastes, and rivers flowing through towns and cities were little better than open sewers of human waste and garbage. This water killed people. Many people. King Leopold of Belgium, when dining with King William of England in the 1830s, reportedly gave great offense by requesting water. "What's that you are drinking, sir?" William asked. "Water, sir," replied Leopold, to which William replied "God damn it, sir, why do you not drink wine? I never allow anyone to drink water at my table."9 While King William may have wanted to show off the quality of his wine cellars, there was also a practical reason for his concern. There was no simple, fast, and reliable way to detect invisible, tasteless, disease-causing contaminants, and a royal host certainly didn't want distinguished guests getting ill at his table.

It was also widely known that water could be made safe—or at least safer—by mixing it with wine or alcohol in concentrations that killed some of the bacteria, or by boiling it and making beer. Hence the crisis facing the Pilgrims in December 1620 and the concern of King William two centuries later: in their experience, drinking untreated water from the local streams and rivers could kill them. Even in nineteenth-century London, many hospitals gave their patients beer rather than water. Women drank homemade lemonade, barley water, or "toast water," which also required boiling.

Polluted water kills. Between 1831 and 1833 a massive wave of Asiatic cholera swept over Britain from Scotland to London, claiming over 50,000 lives.10 In 1832, cholera reached New York and killed more than 3,500 people in a city with a population of only 250,000— as if over 100,000 died today. In the 1840s, the disease again surged back and forth across the continents, killing thousands at a time. In 1846, 15,000 people died in and around Mecca from the disease. Cholera reached Moscow in 1847 and then exploded again throughout Europe. In 1849, tens of thousands more died in London, Paris, and other European cities. Ships carried the disease across the Atlantic to the New World via the ports of New York and New Orleans. Five thousand more died in New York as did several thousand in New Orleans. Cholera then traveled up the Mississippi River valley, spreading by boat to villages and towns. Ten thousand people died in St. Louis and Chicago, and the disease then moved out along the Oregon Trail to the West Coast (an historical fact my children learned when playing the "Oregon Trail" computer game, which would tell them, "The wagon tipped over while you were fording the river. You lose two wagon wheels and little Billy died of cholera."). In California and the Pacific Northwest the contagion merged with more cholera brought down by fur traders from Russia through Alaska. President James Polk is reported to have contracted cholera while in New Orleans in 1849, and died of the disease just a few months after leaving office.[11] In 1853 and 1854, another massive wave of cholera swept back through Europe and America. Russia was reportedly devastated by a million cholera deaths, and once again thousands died in London.

Yet leading doctors and scientists couldn't agree on how people were getting ill or how best to prevent the transmission of most diseases. The sciences of bacteriology, epidemiology, and immunology were still rudimentary. The prevalent theory of the time was that cholera was transmitted through the air as a contagious mist or miasma. While we now know that cholera and typhoid are caused by water-borne bacteria, in the 1800s microscopes were a relatively recent invention and scientists still had little idea what they were looking at when they peered through them at the vast phantasmagoria of bizarre creatures that could be found in a drop of water.

But things were changing fast. Even in the middle of the nineteenth century, new tools of observation, statistics, and epidemiology were being tested, and there were more and more clues that the problem was bad water. Everyone knew that the Thames River flowing through London was dirty. In the 1850s the river smelled so bad on hot summer days that Parliament would adjourn because of the stink. Health officials in England had observed that cholera and typhoid mortality were five to six times higher in the poorer districts getting water from the sewage-contaminated Lower Thames compared to wealthier West London, which received cleaner water from upstream. In 1848 the Lambeth Water Company, one of several private water companies supplying London, moved its water intake upstream on the Thames, above the worst of the sewage discharges, reducing illness in its service area.

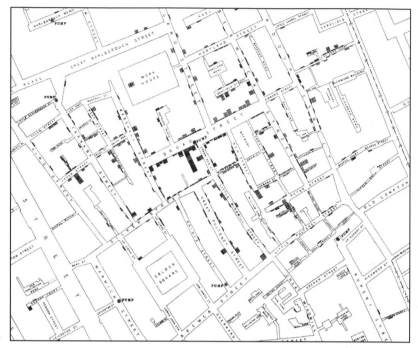

Dr. John Snow's map showing London residences affected by cholera outbreak, and the Broad Street pump, 1854. (From *On the Mode of Communication of Cholera*, 2nd ed. [London: John Churchill, 1855].)

In a now legendary 1854 experiment, Dr. John Snow, a London physician, conducted a simple yet brilliant test that helped to settle the debate about the transmission of cholera. Snow drew a map of a virulent cholera outbreak in one of the poorest neighborhoods of London—an area served by central wells and no sewage collection. He plotted the homes and numbers of people affected and added the location of the wells that provided water for the hardest-hit neighborhoods. The maps he generated and the interviews he conducted with the families of victims convinced him that the source of contamination was the water from one particular well in Broad Street. He received permission from local authorities to remove the pump handle, which forced residents to go to other, uncontaminated wells for water. Within days, the outbreak subsided.

It would take several more decades before the professional disputes over the actual causes of cholera were to end. The Italian scientist Filippo Pacini identified the bacteria that causes cholera in 1854 and argued that the disease must be transmitted in contaminated water, but his work was largely unknown and ignored until the German physician Robert Koch independently rediscovered the bacillus in 1883. (Pacini was ultimately recognized in 1965 when the international committee on nomenclature honored his discovery by naming the nasty bug *Vibrio cholerae Pacini 1854*.) As science and medicine learned more about the sources and prevention of water-related diseases, a revolution in thinking about water swept through the rapidly industrializing world, leading to sewage systems, innovative water treatment, new piping and distribution investments, and efforts to clean up and protect sources of drinking water.

Of course, the simplest and cheapest approach to providing clean water is to take our water from pristine, unpolluted rivers, lakes, or aquifers and to protect those waters from contamination in the first place. Mother Nature naturally provides us with water that is safe to drink. The hydrologic cycle that we all learn about in elementary school—evaporation, condensation, precipitation, runoff, and back to evaporation—is remarkably good at filtering out bad stuff, and if we protect natural sources, we have to do far less later on to provide safe water.

This is what some of the biggest cities in the world have done and it is why they have some of the best tap water. New York City is a classic example. Starting in the mid-1800s—after over a hundred years of political infighting, outbreaks of cholera and other diseases, failed efforts by private companies, and financial missteps—the city built a massive public water system that takes water from protected lands upstate and moves it through huge aqueducts, tunnels, and pipelines to satisfy the needs of more than eight million people living in one of the most densely populated cities in the world. This water is so pure that it receives only minimal treatment even today, though suburban development, rural agricultural activities, and other human disturbances threaten to contaminate the waters at the source.

Cleaning Up Our Water

One of the first steps to purifying water is to use filters to remove suspended particles such as silt, dirt, and other large contaminants. Different kinds of filters, ranging from simple screens to microfiltration, ultrafiltration, and nanofiltration, can remove different sizes and kinds of contaminants. Microfiltration is a low-cost, low-pressure approach to removing suspended solids and fairly large particles down to around 0.1 microns in size and is typically used to clarify dirty water and remove small living organisms. (A "micron" is a millionth of a meter. A strand of human hair is typically around 100 microns in diameter; many bacteria are in the range of a tenth of a micron to ten microns in diameter, though there are larger and smaller ones. Viruses are even smaller.) Ultrafiltration (UF) membranes use higher pressures and smaller pore sizes to separate particulate matter from water. UF membranes typically can remove all bacteria, viruses, and silt in the range of a tenth to a thousandth of a micron. Nanofiltration membranes use even smaller pore sizes and are capable of removing most organic substances, dissolved salts, sugars, metals, and color. Reverse osmosis membranes are the most effective at removing all contaminants down to some of the smallest ions dissolved in water, thus producing remarkably high-quality freshwater, but devoid of most minerals and taste. Indeed, most water produced by reverse osmosis systems has to be re-mixed with minerals or other water in order to be used for drinking.

continued

Problems arise when we introduce bad stuff into the natural hydrologic cycle or fail to clean our water before we use it. Even as we got better and better at filtering and treating water for consumption, modern industrial society got better at dumping bad things into lakes, rivers, and streams. One of the most effective technologies ever developed to contaminate large amounts of water quickly is, ironically, the flush toilet. But in addition to being fouled with basic sewage, water systems also end up as complex stews of industrial and agricultural chemicals and all kinds of other dissolved pollutants.

If the quality of the source water isn't kept pure, we have to clean it up. More and more cities and towns have lost the fight to protect the quality of their source water and now have to rely on sophisticated technologies to remove chemicals, viruses, bacteria,

Cleaning Up Our Water, *continued*

In addition to filtering water, some treatment facilities also sterilize it to kill any remaining organisms that either escaped filtration or were reintroduced in other parts of the process. Among the most common sterilization methods are chlorination, ozonation, and ultraviolet (UV) light treatment. Treating water with chlorine is an old form of sterilization, first used in the late 1800s and throughout the 1900s because it has the excellent property of continuing to kill bacteria along long distribution pipelines. Without some persistent sterilization, clean water put into dirty pipes at the treatment plant can pick up new contaminants on the way to the end user. A drawback to chlorine is that it leaves a slight taste or odor that some people dislike. It is also not very effective against protozoans like *Giardia lamblia* and *Cryptosporidium*, and it can be a nasty material for water managers to handle. Ultraviolet and ozone purification do not alter the taste of the water, but they do not linger in the water or provide a residual sterilizing effect. Ultraviolet radiation is capable of inactivating all types of bacteria and disinfects without the use of heat or chemical additives. The percentage of microorganisms destroyed depends on the intensity of the UV light and the length of time the water is in contact with the radiation. Ozone is a strong oxidizing agent that effectively kills bacteria and protozoa, but like UV, it also has no residual sterilizing power. In the right combinations, these technologies can turn the worst, most polluted waste water into clean, safe drinking water.

---

metals, and other contaminants that get into our water. Indeed, water-treatment systems can be designed to produce the purest drinking water around out of truly horrible water, and almost all such systems are imitations of the natural processes of nature.

Consider how we deal with water purification. Engineered water-treatment systems that flocculate, coagulate, precipitate, condense, and distill water are simply mechanical imitations of natural processes. We build massive sand, charcoal, or mechanical filters that mimic the purification role played by soils. We run water through sophisticated membranes that imitate the ability of cells to separate salts and other things from solution. We stream water past high-intensity ultraviolet lamps that replicate the sterilizing effects of the sun. We grow vats of waste-eating bacteria that take the biological products we excrete and consume them, producing fertilizer, oxygen, and energy. We use fossil fuels to distill water in massive boilers and condensers that are concentrated mechanical reproductions of the hydrologic cycle. All of these artificial interventions are necessary because the population of the planet has outgrown nature's ability to purify our wastes and to provide adequate clean water for our needs. And when our cities began to introduce these water purification technologies, we witnessed the most dramatic and rapid improvements in public health ever achieved.

In the United States in 1900, typhoid, cholera, and water-related diarrheal diseases still caused 200 out of every 100,000 deaths. In late September 1908, Jersey City, New Jersey, became the first major U.S. city to chlorinate its drinking water in an effort to reduce the rates of typhoid and cholera. The health benefits were immediate and other cities rapidly followed suit. By 1920, most U.S. cities were

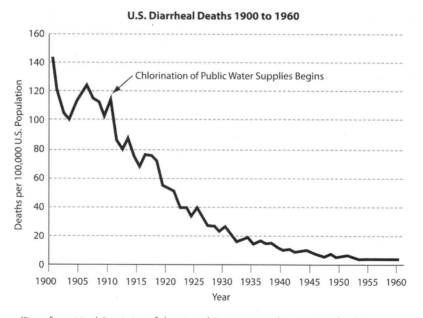

(Data from *Vital Statistics of the United States: Mortality, 1945*, Federal Security Agency, U.S. Public Health Service, Part 1, 1947. Also, *Vital Statistics of the United States: Mortality, 1963*, U.S. Dept. of Health, Education, and Welfare, 1963.)

chlorinating their municipal water supplies. Demographers David Cutler and Grant Miller argue that these innovations in the provision of clean drinking water led to the most rapid improvements in the nation's health ever achieved. They estimate that half of the entire decline in urban death rates and three-quarters of the drop in infant mortality from 1900 to 1940 resulted from the improvement in water quality.[12] Perhaps even more important, the dramatic drop in illness almost certainly contributed to the increase in labor productivity, industrial output, and attendance at school that occurred at the beginning of the twentieth century and helped the United States become the dominant industrial power of the time. By the middle of the century, water-related diseases had dropped by over 95 percent and they have continued to decline.

Water quality in the United States took another huge step forward with the environmental revolution in the 1960s and 1970s. In the late 1960s, accumulated sewage, pollution, oils, and trash were killing our lakes and rivers, like the Cuyahoga River flowing through Cleveland, Ohio. Lake Erie was a cesspool, described by the comedian and talk-show host Johnny Carson as "the place fish go to die." Daily stories about our deteriorating water resources added urgency to the drive for stronger federal oversight over our worsening environment, and in 1970 the U.S. Environmental Protection Agency (EPA) was created to centralize and standardize inconsistent federal and state laws for environmental protection. That same year, Congress passed the Clean Air Act, followed in 1972 by the Clean Water Act, and in 1974 by the federal Safe Drinking Water Act (SDWA).[13]

The Clean Water Act reduced uncontrolled dumping of wastes into surface waters, and the SDWA is the law that requires the U.S. EPA to protect tap water quality. To do so, the EPA sets health-based standards for naturally occurring and human-made contaminants that might be found in our water supplies, and it oversees the water agencies, municipalities, and states that implement the standards. The SDWA sets additional rules for monitoring and for what water providers must do if contamination is found, and it created guidelines for adding limits on new contaminants over time. While the SDWA is urgently in need of improvements, it still requires some of the strongest monitoring and enforcement of tap water quality anywhere, and it is a model for safe water regulation around the world. And what happened when these laws were passed? We learned to trust our tap water . . . at least for a while.

Despite this, as we enter the twenty-first century there is plenty of evidence that tap water, even in parts of the United States, isn't as safe as it could be. Investments in maintaining and improving water systems are falling behind the need. Cities and rural communities are under-investing in replacing old pipes and upgrading treatment plants. The gross failure of our regulatory agencies to monitor and enforce existing standards, and to regularly review and strengthen those standards based on new science, also causes serious and unnecessary problems. Sometimes technological failures permit contaminated water to temporarily enter a municipal distribution system. Combined urban sewer and storm water systems often overflow with sewage during severe storms, dumping untreated wastes into neighboring water bodies. And many people live in houses, towns, or regions that don't have centralized water treatment systems at all, relying instead on local wells or other untreated or marginally treated sources. New monitoring technologies can now detect very low concentrations of contaminants and can identify the presence of new pollutants with unknown public health consequences, but our laws to control these contaminants are badly in need of reform. Thus, water-quality problems inevitably arise, and when they happen and are discovered, we hear about them.

My computer is set to feed me headlines concerning problems with municipal water systems around the world, and those headlines come in daily. Here are just a few examples of stories gleaned from the Internet in the middle of the summer of 2008:

- "The Mississippi Department of Health issues a boil water alert for two counties in the state."
- "DeKalb County [Georgia] Boil Water Alert."

- "West Melbourne, Florida, boil water alert remains in effect today."
- "Residents in west Limerick [Ireland] are being urged to boil their water before drinking it."
- "Tests earlier this week revealed the presence of total coliform bacteria in the [Portland, Connecticut] town's water system, and residents are being urged to use bottled water for drinking and to boil the water for all other uses."
- "23 local government water supply systems in Tasmania operated with a permanent boil water alert during the reporting period."
- "Residents in parts of Norristown, East Norriton, and Plymouth Township [Pennsylvania] should boil their water before drinking after a water main broke early yesterday."
- "Residents in central Hawke's Bay [New Zealand] have been told to boil their drinking water until further notice."
- "The contamination of a water supply that left more than 250,000 people without clean drinking water was blamed today on a small rabbit. Anglian Water [England] said its water treatment works at Pitsford was infected with cryptosporidium, a parasite which causes diarrhoea, after the rabbit found its way into a water tank."[14]

Yuck. Is it any wonder that public doubts about the safety of tap water are growing? If we once again fear our tap water, we will once again look for alternatives we can trust. It's no surprise that the bottled water industry has moved to capitalize upon, and even deepen, these doubts in the minds of consumers. But is bottled water any better or safer? What rules do bottlers have to follow in order to keep their product clean? And who makes them follow those rules?

CHAPTER 3

Selling Unwholesome Provisions

Bottled water's consistent safety and quality is due in part to the extensive FDA requirements, individual state regulations, and industry standards which bottled water must meet. All of these combine to make bottled water one of the safest food products available for human consumption.
— International Bottled Water Association[1]

Water bottling is one of the least regulated industries in the U.S.— much less regulated than our public tap water. Scientific studies even show that bottled water is no safer than tap water, and can sometimes be less safe . . .
— Corporate Accountability International[2]

Look at these two statements carefully. Confused? Me too, and I've read and reread the rules about protecting both bottled water and tap water. As we saw all too clearly with the crisis that overwhelmed our global financial systems in 2008 and 2009, the problem is often not the lack of laws and regulations. The problem is that the rules we have are complicated and contradictory, full of loopholes and ambiguity. They vary from country to country or state to state, and they are weakly applied and rarely enforced. This doesn't make for consumer confidence about water quality no matter what you choose to drink. And confusion about water quality opens the door to competing and conflicting claims over safety, and worse, to actual contamination and health risks.

Protecting water quality and the quality of the goods sold to the public requires clear and consistent standards. Even our founding fathers understood the need for laws to protect against contaminated food and drink. On March 8, 1785, the Massachusetts legislature passed one of my all-time favorite pieces of legislation: "An Act against selling unwholesome provisions." In a few short words they describe the problems and lay out the recommended punishment.

"Whereas some evilly disposed persons, from motives of avarice and filthy lucre, have been induced to sell diseased, corrupted, contagious or unwholesome provisions, to the great nuisance of public health and peace: Be it therefore enacted by the Senate and House of Representatives . . . That if any person shall sell any such diseased, corrupted, contagious or unwholesome provisions, whether for meat or drink, knowing the same without making it known to the buyer . . . he shall be punished by fine, imprisonment, standing in the pillory, and binding to the good behavior, or one or more of these punishments, to be inflicted according to the degree and aggravation of the offense."3

Nearly two hundred years later, the public is still threatened with "corrupted, contagious, or unwholesome provisions" sold with "motives of avarice and filthy lucre" to "the great nuisance of public health and peace." And perhaps there hasn't been enough "imprisonment, standing in the pillory, and binding to the good behaviour" for such "evilly disposed persons."

In the United States, national water-quality laws have been in place in one form or another for many decades, and provide at least a foundation for protecting public health. In a peculiar twist, however, the federal agencies given oversight over our drinking water have no authority over bottled water—a product never anticipated by the drafters of the original federal drinking water laws. Instead, the U.S. Food and Drug Administration (FDA) regulates bottled water because it is considered a "food product" sold in individual containers. This also explains the presence of the remarkably uninformative "Nutrition Label" found on U.S. bottled water, which carefully, and

> ## An Act againſt ſelling unwholeſome Proviſions.
>
> *WHEREAS* ſome evilly diſpoſed perſons, from motives of avarice and fil-
> thy lucre, have been induced to ſell diſeaſed, corrupted, contagious or un-
> wholeſome proviſions, to the great nuiſance of public health and peace :
>
> Be it therefore enacted by the Senate and Houſe of Repreſentatives, in Ge-
> neral Court aſſembled, and by the authority of the ſame, That if any perſon
> ſhall ſell any ſuch diſeaſed, corrupted, contagious or unwholeſome pro-
> viſions, whether for meat or drink, knowing the ſame without making
> it known to the buyer, and being thereof convicted before the Juſtices
> of the General Seſſions of the Peace, in the county where ſuch offence
> ſhall be committed, or the Juſtices of the Supreme Judicial Court, he
> ſhall be puniſhed by fine, impriſonment, ſtanding in the pillory, and
> binding to the good behaviour, or one or more of theſe puniſhments,
> to be inflicted according to the degree and aggravation of the offence.
>
> [This act paſſed March 8, 1785.]

Perhaps the earliest piece of U.S. consumer-protection
legislation, Massachusetts, 1785.

uselessly, lists no calories, no fat, no sodium, no protein, no vitamins, and no carbs. Bottlers must also comply with additional food
regulations, such as those that govern packaging facilities,[4] and the
Public Health Security and Bioterrorism Preparedness and Response
Act of 2002 (Bioterrorism Act).[5]

Officially, the FDA's bottled water standards are supposed to be
no less protective of the public health than the EPA's regulations for
public drinking water.[6] Indeed, while bottled-water quality standards
are, for the most part, similar to our tap water standards, they are
not identical. Some of the differences are minor or inconsequential.
Some are potentially significant. And the different regulatory structures and authorities mean that there are ambiguities, differences in
standards and practices, and loopholes big enough to encourage (or
at least to fail to discourage) "evilly disposed persons."

The ambiguities in regulations have been used to bolster safety
claims on both sides of the bottled water debate. In 2008, Kim Jeffries,
President and CEO of Nestlé Water, said:

> Frankly, there is no comparison between the two products: tap
> water and bottled water. While the regulatory standards are
> almost identical to be protective of public health, bottled water

has more control over the quality of the groundwater sources used (in the case of spring water), much more highly specialized treatment, and does not need to add chlorine as a disinfectant. The bottle itself locks in the quality so the consumer gets quality assurance in every bottle.[7]

At the other end of the spectrum of opinion, bottled water opponents regularly lament the inadequacies of bottled water quality regulations. Corporate Accountability International, an advocacy group that runs an aggressive public campaign against bottled water, tells us, "Water bottling is one of the least regulated industries in the U.S.— much less regulated than our public tap water. Scientific studies even show that bottled water is no safer than tap water, and can sometimes be less safe, containing elevated levels of arsenic, bacteria, and other contaminants."[8]

Where does the truth lie? Perhaps not surprisingly, somewhere between these two extreme positions. There have been some efforts to reconcile the EPA and FDA water standards but important differences remain. Whenever the EPA issues a new regulation for a drinking water contaminant or requires a change in method for treating a contaminant, the FDA has around half a year to either adopt a comparable standard or "make a finding" that the contaminant is not in water used for bottling. But both the EPA and the FDA have been slow to identify new contaminants in drinking water and to regulate them, and they seem unable to plug several big loopholes.

Here's one such loophole: while U.S. drinking water standards apply to all municipal tap water, FDA regulations only apply to food products sold in interstate commerce, leaving a vast amount of bottled water that never enters "interstate commerce" without consistent protection. By some estimates, this loophole alone exempts 60 to 70 percent of all bottled water from federal regulations.[9] Conversely, some FDA bottled-water standards are more stringent than EPA's public drinking-water standards. EPA standards for lead in tap water are set at 15 parts per billion; the FDA has set them at only 5 parts per billion for bottled water because it is easier to keep lead out of bottled water than water delivered through piping systems to a home.

Some states, but not all, also regulate bottled water. Many states have bottled water rules that are as comprehensive, or in some instances even stricter, than the FDA's, yet ten states don't regulate bottled water at all. In general, states are responsible under federal law for inspecting and approving water sources, certifying testing laboratories, and performing inspections of bottled water plants. Bottlers that sell their products in other states are subject to periodic, unannounced inspections by the FDA, but such inspections are very rare. Moreover, these inspections almost never test bottled water *quality*; the FDA typically just looks to see that bottlers are in compliance with other kinds of regulations.

Perhaps the most significant and worrisome difference between the EPA and FDA standards for water is the standard for coliform bacteria, especially *E. coli* and fecal bacteria. Coliforms are bacteria found in human and animal waste, and we do not want them in our drinking water. Of special concern is a form called *Escherichia coli* (or *E. coli*). *E. coli* is hard to detect—especially a subset of *E. coli* that can be deadly. As a result, the EPA has a special regulation called the "Total Coliform Rule" that requires all public water systems to monitor tap water for total coliform, which is easier to find, as a first indicator that there might be something wrong with the water supply. EPA's "Total Coliform Rule" sets the rules for how often community water systems (cities, towns, universities, and other communities with their own water systems) must test for coliform. Systems with fewer than 50,000 customers must test 60 times per month. Systems serving 2.5 million customers or more must test 420 times per month—dozens of times a day. Small systems serving fewer than 1,000 people must only test quarterly.[10]

If there are no "total" coliforms in these tests, then the assumption is that there are no "bad" coliforms. So far so good. But if any coliforms are detected (after a repeat check), the water must then be retested for the more dangerous fecal coliform, *E. coli*. If fecal coliform are found, the state must be notified by the end of the day and action must be taken to disinfect the tap-water system. That's right, public notification is supposed to happen the same day.

The coliform rules for bottled water are much weaker. Under FDA standards, bottled water must only be tested for general coliforms, and only once a week. Furthermore, the FDA standards permit bottled water to contain, depending on the test used, a small number of coliform organisms. If the number of coliform organisms found is below a certain level, there is no additional requirement that the water be tested to see if they are the dangerous kinds, and even more remarkably, there is no requirement that the water be pulled from distribution. Indeed, while any violation of tap water standards is considered grounds for enforcement, bottled water found with coliform can still be sold if the bottles are labeled as "containing excessive bacteria." Finally, there is no requirement that bottlers promptly report any contamination they discover, publicly notify their users of the contamination, or recall the product. And as we'll see shortly, when bottled water is recalled, it is often months after the product went out to consumers—too late to actually protect the public.

In 2008 the FDA proposed strengthening the U.S. standard so that it would be more in line with tap water protections by requiring bottlers that find coliform in the source water or finished product to conduct additional tests for *E. coli*. In proposing these new rules, the FDA admitted what the bottled water industry has long denied: bottled water drinkers are not adequately protected from drinking water with fecal pathogens. "Under current FDA regulations, the potential exists for fecal pathogens in ground water to be undetected and be distributed to consumers in bottled water and cause illness."[11] If bacteria were to be found, the bottlers would have to take actions to stop the contamination, but even the new proposed rules—which are supposed to go into effect in December 2009—have lax monitoring and enforcement mechanisms, weak reporting and disclosure requirements, and, like other federal bottled water regulations, would still not apply to the vast quantities of bottled water that do not enter interstate commerce.[12]

In comparison, again, look at the difference between U.S. and European standards for coliform. The standards imposed by the European Union for bottled spring water are far stricter, requiring that analyses be conducted to demonstrate the "absence of parasites and pathogenic microorganisms" and in particular, the absence of *E. coli*, other coliforms, and fecal streptococci.[13] Without better standards for bottled water, we cannot be sure of what's actually in those bottles. And standards alone aren't enough. No matter how good water-quality standards are—and we've seen that they are, at best, full of loopholes for bottled water—trouble is bound to arise if we don't regularly test and monitor. And we don't. The deeper we look into how bottled water is tested and monitored, the more concerned we should be.

Contaminated by Crickets

You won't find what you don't look for. As Ronald Reagan used to say with regard to arms control negotiations, "Doveryai, no proveryai," or "Trust, but verify." This maxim holds true for arms control and it holds true for contaminants in water. At first glance, there seem to be far fewer problems with bottled water quality in the United States and elsewhere than with the quality of tap water. There are two plausible explanations for this: either it really is safer, or we're ignorant of the true problems with bottled water. In the United States and many other countries the latter is certainly true, which means we don't know if the former is true or not.

The system for testing and monitoring the quality of bottled water is so flawed that we simply have no comprehensive assessment of actual bottled water quality. Don't misunderstand me. The inadequacies of U.S. rules for testing bottled water do not mean that bottled water quality is poor. If bottled water were monitored as consistently, frequently, and accurately as tap water, the evidence might show that it is just as good, or even better on average, than tap water. Given how much consumers pay for it, we certainly have the right to expect it to be better. But we're just not looking. The bad news is that when we do actually look, we find evidence that there are potentially serious quality problems with bottled water, lurking just under the cap. And outside of the United States, where there are often no rules for testing bottled water at all, there is growing evidence that bottled water quality can be terrible.

Any water-quality law is only as good as the frequency of the inspections, the independence of the tests, and the effectiveness of enforcement. On all three counts, bottled water protections are inadequate. In the United States, FDA rules determine how, and how often, bottled water quality is checked, but actual FDA inspections for the purpose of testing water quality are very rare. In fact, most of the FDA inspections that do happen don't involve actually taking and testing of water samples. Rather, inspectors simply evaluate compliance with other rules, such as whether bottlers are analyzing water according to the required schedules—hardly the kind of oversight that inspires confidence in actual bottled water quality. And as noted earlier, bottled water that doesn't enter interstate commerce isn't even subject to the FDA's weak rules and inspections.

Bottled water is a very low priority for FDA inspections partly because the agency believes that "bottled water has a good safety record," and partly because the FDA's overall ability to inspect food production and safety is weak.[14] But this is a circular argument: Bottled water has a good safety record, the FDA says, so there is little need to actually conduct inspections. But without regular independent inspections, actual problems are unlikely to be discovered.

Testing for contamination is left almost entirely to the bottlers themselves. While the FDA specifies approved testing methods, bottlers are not required to use those methods. They may use any other testing method so long as their "bottled water can pass the tests used by FDA in its own laboratories, should testing be performed by the FDA."[15] The FDA also leaves considerable authority to the states and to the bottlers themselves. In particular, the FDA asks states to inspect, sample, analyze, and approve water sources and the final product. But FDA rules on bottled water preempt many state regulations that might be more stringent than federal regulations.[16]

Title 21, part 129, section 35 of the FDA regulations, which specifies details for testing bottled water, states: "Analysis of the sample *may* be performed for the plant by competent commercial laboratories (e.g., Environmental Protection Agency (EPA) and State-certified laboratories)." [Emphasis added.] "May" be performed. Not "must" be performed. Not even "should" be performed. This is pretty weak. Even weaker, analysis of bottled water quality is supposed to be done by "competent commercial laboratories," but if the source of the water is municipal tap water systems, the bottlers can simply substitute public water system testing results, rather than do their own testing.[17]

The FDA requires bottled water plants to analyze source water and finished products once a week for bacteria (if the water comes from a source other than municipal water supply), once a year for most chemical and physical contaminants, and as little as once every four years for radiological contaminants.[18] This frequency of testing is too low to ensure reliable quality or to catch intermittent problems. But even worse, there is no mandatory requirement that the results of bottled water tests be sent to the FDA or that the FDA independently confirm the results. Test results and notices of violations for tap water must be reported to state or federal officials, and municipal water agencies must send all of their customers a comprehensive water-quality report every year. There is no comparable mandatory public reporting for water bottlers. Bottlers are supposed to maintain records of their test results for two years and keep them available for official review "at reasonable times," but they do not have to share them with the consumer.

What actually happens if bottled water is tested and found to contain a substance at a level greater than what is allowed? In the United States, federal rules say that when the microbiological, physical, chemical, or radiological quality of bottled water is below that prescribed in the standard, the label of the bottled water bottle must contain a statement of substandard quality, such as "Contains Excessive Bromate," "Contains Excessive Bacteria," or "Excessively Radioactive."[19] In other words, the bottler is supposed to stop filling bottles, create a new label, and paste it on the contaminated bottles. You can imagine how often this happens. I've never seen or heard of a case where a bottler relabeled a bottle as containing "Excessive" anything.

In 1999 the General Accounting Office (GAO) issued a scathing report that criticized the testing and enforcement actions of the FDA: "The fragmented system was not developed under any rational plan but was patched together over many years to address specific health threats from particular food products." Among the criticisms the GAO offered were "inconsistent and inflexible oversight and enforcement authorities, inefficient resource use, and ineffective coordination."[20] A new GAO study released in June 2009 found that little has been done over the past decade to fix these problems, and food (and bottled water) testing in the United States remains inconsistent, piecemeal, and flawed. Among their findings was that while the FDA does very few actual inspections of water bottlers, the few they conducted between 2000 and 2008 found problems a remarkable 35 percent of the time. Even this warning sign led to "little enforcement action."[21] The GAO also concluded that relying on the states to do the job of protecting bottled water quality was inadequate, that state protections were "less comprehensive than state requirements to safeguard tap water," and that other countries do better: for example, as noted above, European regulations specify that bottled water cannot contain any coliform bacteria. So do Canadian rules. Turkish regulations require inspections of bottled water facilities more frequently than FDA regulations.

"FDA was our country's first consumer protection agency and Americans have relied on FDA to ensure the safety of their food and drugs for 100 years," said Representative Henry A. Waxman, a leading defender of consumer protections in Congress. "Under the [George W.] Bush Administration, FDA has undermined enforcement and betrayed its consumer-first legacy." Similarly, Representative John Dingell, chairman of the House Committee on Energy and Commerce, said in November 2008, "Over the course of our investigation, the committee has found that FDA not only failed in its basic mission, but refused to admit its failures and take steps to protect Americans from unsafe food and drugs."[22] It came as little surprise in March 2009 when President Barack Obama called the U.S. food safety system a "public health hazard." "There are certain things only government can do," President Obama said. "And one of those things is ensuring that the foods we eat, and the medicines we take, are safe and don't cause us harm."[23]

Lax oversight notwithstanding, most of our tap water is completely safe; most of our bottled water is probably completely safe. But to know for sure, we must look carefully. And when we do actually look, we sometimes find more than we bargained for.

Instances of bottled water contamination are rarely reported to the public or media, but such instances are discovered more frequently than we know and probably occur more frequently than we actually discover. When tap water is contaminated, the story is usually carried on the news that evening because water agencies are required to report it to the public and take quick action to correct the problem. Because the frequency of testing for bottled water is much lower and the reporting requirements are less strict, the discovery of contaminated bottled water may occur days or weeks after the product has been delivered to markets and sold—if it is discovered at all. Even more astounding, if bottled water is found to be contaminated, there is no requirement that it be automatically recalled. If contamination is discovered in bottled water, the bottler is required to take actions to "remove or reduce" the contamination but is under no obligation to inform the public or recall the tainted product. And the public notification, if any is even given, may be far too late.

Contrary to what the public might expect, the FDA is not authorized under law to order the recall of contaminated bottled water. In general, the FDA expects companies to take full responsibility for product recalls. The FDA is authorized to prescribe a recall only when a medical device, human tissue products, or contaminated infant formula poses a risk to human health.[24] For other contaminated products, the FDA can only request that a company recall a contaminated product. If the firm refuses, the FDA can then choose to pursue legal actions. These include seizure of available product and asking a court to order the company to recall the product. By this time, of course, the contaminated product is likely to be long gone from the shelves.

Sometimes recalls do occur. If a recall is issued, it falls into one of three classes according to the level of hazard involved:

- Class I recalls are for dangerous or defective products that could cause serious health problems or death.
- Class II recalls are for products that might cause a temporary health problem or pose only a slight threat of a serious nature.
- Class III recalls are for products that are unlikely to cause any adverse health effects, but that violate FDA labeling or manufacturing regulations. Examples for bottled water might be a container defect, bad taste, odd color, a lack of proper labeling, or other flaws that pose no health risks.

The FDA applies different strategies for each type of recall. For the most serious problems, the FDA will usually perform spot checks to make sure that the defective product has been recalled and removed from shelves. In contrast, for a Class III recall, the Agency may take no action to make sure the product is off the market. The company recalling the product may issue a press release, but the FDA rarely seeks publicity about a recall unless a serious public health hazard exists.

Information on actual bottled water recalls is incomplete and very hard to find. How many recalls of bottled water have there been, and for what reasons? One source of information is newspaper accounts, but a systematic search of newspapers reveals only a handful of examples. A better source of information should be the FDA website, where recalls are supposed to be available in a public database called the FDA Enforcement Report Index. Food and drug recalls are listed by year going back to 1995. Pre-1995 recalls are available in a separate file. When I used the FDA search engine to find "bottled water" recalls, only around a dozen results came up. If the search is done without the quotation marks, 33 results come up but many of these have nothing to do with bottled water products (they include, for example, products bottled in water).

In order to find all of the public recalls of bottled water in the FDA database, one must search inside every individual weekly report. I did this going back to 1990 and discovered that many bottled water recalls occurred but are not found by the FDA search engines. All told, I found nearly a hundred actual bottled water recalls.

Even worse, it turns out that not all recalls of bottled water are actually listed in the database. How did I discover this? When I began my detailed search, I knew of a recall that was not listed by the FDA. In December 2005 I had seen a small news story about a recall of Ethos Spring Water, posted on the Starbucks website. I was familiar with Ethos—a brand of bottled water started by two young entrepreneurs hoping to use the concept of bottled water as a way to raise awareness, and money, to help bring safe water to developing countries. Their initial effort had attracted the attention, and then the financing, of Starbucks, which had recently purchased the company and expanded its market. Even today, you can buy Ethos Water at most Starbucks, and a part of the money generated is donated to water projects around the world. (I describe Ethos in more detail later in this book.)

In early December 2005 the company discovered excessive levels of bromate—a potential carcinogen—in their water, which was bottled by the Chameleon Beverage Company for distribution in the western United States. To their credit, Starbucks initiated a voluntary recall right away, changed bottling companies, and posted a story about it on their own website. Yet when I checked with the FDA, this recall was not listed in the official database, even eight months later. Moreover, Chameleon Beverage Company made bottled water for other companies under contract but none of them ever announced a recall and FDA never required one. Hmm, I thought, if this one recall wasn't listed, could there be others?

In late February 2006 I filed a Freedom of Information Act (FOIA) request with the FDA for a list of all bottled water recalls not listed in their website database. Two months later, I received "full access" to their list of additional recalls—a total of only five, including one recalled for high coliforms and another for glass particles. Yet once again, the Ethos recall was not included. I knew that Ethos had reported their recall to the FDA, so I filed an FOIA appeal in April 2006, indicating that I knew of additional recalls not publicly listed on the website and also not released in their first response to my request. This request produced an additional, larger set of recalls, including the Ethos incident. This information, together with the publicly available data, suggest that there have been over 100 incidents of bottled water contamination leading to recalls, a third of which have never been made public.[25]

The first recall on this list is perhaps the most famous one of all. In February 1990 the leading bottled water brand on the planet at the time, Perrier, was discovered to have excessive levels of benzene. As might be expected, given lax federal testing and monitoring, the contamination was not discovered by the FDA but by the Environmental Health Department in Mecklenburg County, North Carolina. The Department was using Perrier water as their standard in the lab for testing other waters because they assumed it was consistently pure. When they began seeing problems in all of their water-quality tests, they cleaned their lab, recalibrated equipment, and redid their tests before realizing that the contamination was coming from the Perrier they were buying at the local store. Upon testing the Perrier itself, they found levels of benzene that violated federal standards, and they alerted the FDA.

The first reaction by Perrier was to deny that there was any health risk. "A cup of non-freeze-dried coffee contains more benzene," a company representative told the *Economist* magazine.[26]

They then attributed the problem to a faulty machine serving only the North American market, and as public pressure grew they began recalling bottles sold in the United States. More independent tests, however, discovered that the problem affected their entire global production for the previous six months, leading to the complete recall of millions of bottles and more bad press. Even today, the actions of the company around the discovery, the piecemeal recall, the publicity, and a botched relaunch of the product later in 1991 are considered textbook examples of how not to conduct a recall when a product is discovered to be tainted. Michael White, in his 2002 book *A Short Course in International Marketing Blunders*, reports that in 1991 Perrier's share of the bottled water market in the United States dropped from 13 percent to 8 percent; in the United Kingdom it dropped from a massive 49 percent to 30 percent; and it even dropped substantially in France.[27] The ultimate cost to the company was hundreds of millions of dollars and substantial consumer goodwill. As Andre Soltner, owner of Lutèce, the famous French restaurant in Manhattan, said upon hearing that Perrier was contaminated with benzene, "Oh my God. Maybe we'll sell some wine now."[28]

The Perrier contamination example is fascinating, but it is not the only one. The full list of bottled water recalls issued in the United States alone, even under a regulatory system that doesn't require careful monitoring, reporting, or recalls of contaminated bottled water, includes a remarkable list of contaminants. In addition to benzene, bottles have been found to contain mold, sodium hydroxide, kerosene, styrene, algae, yeast, tetrahydrofuran, sand, fecal coliforms and other forms of bacteria, elevated chlorine, "filth," glass particles, sanitizer, and, in my very favorite example, crickets.

Yes, crickets. In May 1994 a bottler in Nacogdoches, Texas, issued a recall for sparkling water found to be contaminated with crickets. The water was distributed in Alabama, Florida, and Georgia, and the recall notice wasn't issued until seven months later in December 1994, making it unlikely that consumers were notified in time to avoid buying the contaminated bottles.

This delay between the discovery of contamination and public notification is another serious flaw with the entire recall system. Even when recalls are publicly posted by the FDA to their website, the notice can come months—often many months—after the contamination has been discovered and long after the water has been sold and consumed. Unless there is prompt media attention in the market where the contaminated water is being sold, and prompt voluntary action by the company itself, the water is unlikely to be kept out of the hands—and stomachs—of consumers. In July 1993 over 24,000 bottles of spring water in Virginia were discovered to be contaminated with mold, but the recall didn't occur until September. In February 1994 nearly 20,000 cases of spring water from Washington State, distributed nationwide, were also contaminated with mold, but the public recall didn't come until June. Over 7,000 gallons of purified drinking water from a Tennessee bottler, distributed in six Southern states, were discovered contaminated with fecal coliforms in August 1994, but the recall didn't come until October. More than a million bottles of spring water from New York, distributed throughout the northeastern United States between March and October 1995, were found to have mold, but no recall was initiated until May of the following year. Nearly 20,000 gallons of bottled drinking water from a dairy in Michigan were found to contain sanitizer with peroxyacic acid in August 2001, but the recall didn't go out until March 2002, seven months later. In September 2008 Nestlé Pure Life water containing diluted cleaning solution was recalled. According to the notice, the water was distributed in Connecticut, New York, Delaware, New Jersey, and Pennsylvania three months earlier. The list goes on and on.

Problems with bottled water quality are not limited to the United States. In fact, the harder we look, the more we find. Countries with inadequate regulation and monitoring inevitably have problems with water quality and contamination. Even countries with good regulatory systems find contamination in bottled water, and many developing countries have no bottled water regulation at all. A comprehensive survey conducted in Ireland in 2007 found that 7 percent of the samples of bottled water tested were contaminated with something that exceeded Irish or European Union guidelines, more than 6 percent of the water had coliform bacteria, and some samples had *E. coli*—the worst form of fecal contamination.[29] Equally disturbing, the Irish Food Safety Authority admitted that they had shared the results of their survey with the industry but still had not formally released it to the public a year later. Some bottled waters were withdrawn from sale but no public notification was ever made, and the companies violating standards were never named.[30]

Ireland's experience with bottled water is not unique. A study done in the Netherlands in 2004 tested 68 commercial mineral waters, one tap water, and one sample from a natural well, taken from a total of sixteen different countries. Overall, 40 percent of the samples had contamination with bacteria or fungus.[31] In 2003, eleven brands of mineral water were declared contaminated and unfit for human consumption by the Pakistan Council of Research on Water Resources (PCRWR), yet a year later they were still available for sale in markets.[32] In 2006 Indonesian police closed down a company that recovered plastic bottles from the local garbage dump, filled them with local groundwater, relabeled them, and sold them.[33] Thirty-nine primary school children were poisoned by bottled water contaminated by paraffin in Ho Chi Minh City, Vietnam.[34] Sanitation officers in Manila, Philippines, warned residents to beware of unsafe water from bottled water filling shops operating with no permits.[35]

Unsafe water, from any source, can make people sick. Whether water is provided by public agencies or private companies, it must be carefully and strictly regulated. Too often, in too many places around the world, such oversight is lacking. But even U.S. regulations concerning bottled water, because they are neither sufficiently strict nor adequately enforced, sometimes offer no greater consumer protection in the United States than if there were no regulations at all.

If people are going to buy bottled water because they believe it to be clean and safe, regulatory agencies responsible for protecting public health must do more to ensure that it really is clean and safe. At present, customers have no such assurances.

CHAPTER 4

If It's Called "Arctic Spring," Why Is It from Florida?

Calories, 0; Fat, 0; Cholesterol, 0; Sodium, 0;
Total Carbohydrate, 0; Protein, 0.
— Typical information on a bottled water
label in the United States

"Alaska Premium Glacier Drinking Water: Pure Glacier Water from the
Last Unpolluted Frontier" was actually drawn from Public Water System
#111241 in Juneau.
— Brian Howard, *E—The Environmental Magazine*[1]

ONCE UPON A TIME, when you bought Poland Spring bottled
water it actually came from the famous Poland Spring in the state of
Maine. Today, Poland Spring is no longer a "source" but a "brand."
The water in the bottle might come from Poland Spring, or it might
come from Clear Spring, Evergreen Spring, Spruce Spring, Garden
Spring, Bradford Spring, or White Cedar Spring—other Maine
water sources owned by Nestlé Waters North America. There is no
way to know. And Nestlé isn't saying.

Poland Spring water has a long history. In 1845 the Ricker family began to bottle local spring water. They sold it in grocery stores in
clay jugs—three gallons for 15 cents—and wooden barrels to sea

captains and other travelers. By 1860 claims of health benefits, paid advertisements, and word of mouth had increased sales substantially, and Poland Spring water was being sold as far away as "the Deep South and the Far West." In 1895 the water won top honors "over all the other waters of the world" at the Chicago World's Fair. It won the Grand Prize for water at the 1904 St. Louis World's Fair, and the Ricker family went on to build bottling houses and a major resort that hosted celebrities such as Mae West, U.S. presidents Cleveland and Taft, and business leaders. Demand continued to grow throughout the twentieth century, putting more and more pressure on the limited flow of the original spring. There were rumors that the spring stopped flowing in 1967 because of excessive pumping of the groundwater feeding the spring.[2] In 1980 The Perrier Group, later to become Nestlé Waters North America, purchased Poland Spring as one of their flagship brands, which also include Perrier and Arrowhead Spring. By the early 2000s sales of Poland Spring water exceeded $600 million a year and the demand for water had skyrocketed. In order to keep up, Nestlé had to find other sources of supply, and the name "Poland Spring" became a "brand" rather than a specific source.

Not all consumers were happy with the change. A class-action lawsuit filed in Connecticut Superior Court in 2003 contended that Nestlé was guilty of false advertising by implying on their labels that the water comes from Poland Spring.[3] The suit alleged that the production of Poland Spring depends on source wells drawing more than six million gallons of water a year, none of which comes from the original Poland Spring, and some of which are vulnerable to surface contamination. Similar suits were filed in Massachusetts and New Jersey Superior Courts. Without admitting to any wrongdoing, in September 2003 Nestlé Waters agreed to settle this class-action suit, step up quality control, and pay $10 million over five years in discounts to consumers and contributions to charities—but there was no requirement that they clarify their labels.[4] In 2009 I asked a representative of the company what fraction, if any, of Poland Spring water now comes from the actual Poland Spring, how much Arrow-head Spring water is in Arrowhead brand bottled water, and how much real Perrier Spring water is in the Perrier brand bottled water? After several months and communications, as this book was going to press, the company had still refused to release this information.

What is really in the water bottles we buy? We know, or hope, that it is water, but it turns out we rarely know what kind of water it is, or precisely where it comes from, even if it has a famous name or historical association. We assume—perhaps mistakenly—that it is clean and safe to drink, but we don't know how it was treated, who tested it, or what the results were. We want it to taste good, but we aren't told details of the mineral composition, which determines the actual taste.

All we know is what we're told on the label, and what we're told on the label in the United States is minimal and misleading. What might a good water bottle tell you? Should it clearly and honestly describe what kind of water is actually in the bottle? Which spring or municipal system the water comes from? What kind of purifica-tion treatment, if any, it has received? Should the label accurately specify the detailed mineral composition of the water, which affects the taste? And finally, what if labels told the consumer where to go to get up-to-date information about where to see detailed water-quality tests, to ask for more information, or to file complaints?

Current bottled water labeling laws in the United States require none of these things. There are rules in the U.S. about some of these things, but these rules are inconsistent and inconsistently applied, and bottled water labels often do more to conceal information than reveal it. In order to provide at least some help for consumers, the U.S. Food and Drug Administration is supposed to oversee a set of labeling rules that apply to some (though not all) of the bottled water sold in the United States. First of all, the FDA defines bottled water as "water that is intended for human consumption and that is sealed in bottles or other containers with no added ingredients except that it may optionally contain safe and suitable antimicrobial agents." So no added ingredients. ("Vitamin waters" and other "enhanced" water drinks are considered to be more akin to carbonated soft drinks or fruit drinks.)

The FDA further restricts the names that can be used to describe the water—not the commercial brand name, but how the kind of water itself is to be identified.[5] This name is called the "identity." According to the Federal Food, Drug, and Cosmetic Act (FFDCA): "A bottled water product must meet the appropriate Standard of Identity and bear the required name on its label or it may be deemed misbranded under the FFDCA."[6]

The most common Standards of Identity are shown in the box on the next page. But don't expect these names to offer much enlightenment. Despite, or maybe because of, the great diversity of these "identities," the average buyer is unlikely to understand the differences among "distilled," "deionized," and "purified," or among "well," "spring," ground," and "artesian" water. And consumers deserve to know much more.

In contrast to U.S. labeling requirements, the European Community requires that labels on natural mineral waters and spring waters sold in Europe include the following mandatory information:

(a) A statement of the analytical composition, giving its characteristic constituents,

(b) The place where the spring is exploited and the name of the spring, and

(c) Information on any treatments used to process the water before bottling.[7]

The failure to provide clear labels on U.S. bottled water leads to consumer confusion. Arrowhead Spring Water, for example, also bottled by Nestlé, used to come from the actual Arrowhead springs on the slopes of the San Bernardino mountains, but now, like "Poland Spring," it is just a brand name for water that comes from many different springs across southern California. Nestlé has even

U.S. "Standards of Identity" for U.S. Bottled Waters

"**Artesian water**" or "artesian well water" is water from a well tapping a confined aquifer in which the water level stands at some height above the top of the aquifer. Artesian water may be collected with the assistance of external force to enhance the natural underground pressure.

"**Ground water**" includes water from a subsurface saturated zone that is under a pressure equal to or greater than atmospheric pressure. Ground water "must not" be under the direct influence of surface water as defined by the U.S. Environmental Protection Agency (EPA),* though determining "direct influence" is dicey, at best, as I discuss later.

"**Mineral water**" is water containing not less than 250 parts per million (ppm) total dissolved solids (TDS), coming from a source tapped at one or more bore holes or springs, originating from a geologically and physically protected underground water source. No minerals may be added to this water. If the TDS content is below 500 ppm, the label is supposed to say "low mineral content"; if the TDS content is above 1,500 ppm, the label should read "high mineral content." There is no requirement to list the individual minerals or their concentrations.

"**Purified water**" is water that has been has been treated by distillation, deionization, reverse osmosis, or other "suitable processes," and that meets the definition of "purified water" in the United States Pharmacopeia (twenty-third revision). Major bottlers like Coca-Cola, PepsiCo, Nestlé, and others produce and sell "purified water" that often originates from municipal water systems.

"**Sparkling bottled water**" is water that, after treatment and possible artificial replacement of carbon dioxide, contains the same level of carbon dioxide as water directly from the source.

"**Spring water**" is water derived from an underground formation from which water flows naturally to the surface of the earth. Spring water is to be collected only at the spring or through a bore hole tapping the underground formation directly feeding the spring.

"**Sterile water**" is water that meets the requirements under the "Sterility Test" in the Twenty-Third Revision of the United States Pharmacopeia.

"**Well water**" is water from a hole bored, drilled, or otherwise constructed in the ground, which taps the water of an aquifer.

---

* In the Code of Federal Regulations, 40 CFR 141.2

---

proposed tapping a spring in Colorado and calling it Arrowhead.[8] Consumers no longer know the specific source of the water in the bottle they buy or if it is from a mix of sources.

Even when the water comes from a municipal water supply, which is increasingly the case, the bottler does not have to state which one, or describe whether or not the water goes through additional processing. Coca-Cola's Dasani, PepsiCo's Aquafina, and Nestlé's Pure Life brands come from dozens of different bottling plants, which treat local municipal waters so they all taste the same. If you buy Dasani in the San Francisco Bay Area, you're probably getting water bottled at their plant in San Leandro. Buy Dasani in southern Michigan and it probably originated as municipal water in Detroit. But the bottlers don't have to say and they often package their bottle in a way to draw on the cachet of spring water.

Until mid-2007 bottles of Aquafina offered no indication that the water originates from local tap water systems, and even today it has a lovely logo designed like a mountain range. Curious consumers might have seen a small "P.W.S." on the label, but until advocacy groups pressured the company to actually spell out "public water source," most consumers probably had no idea that they were drinking reprocessed tap water. In announcing the change, PepsiCo spokeswoman Michelle Naughton spun, "If this helps clarify the fact that the water originates from public sources, then it's a reasonable thing to do."[9] At the same time that PepsiCo announced their intention to modify their labels, Nestlé announced it would be changing its labels to "identify the source of the water, whether it's from a municipal supply or ground-water well source."

Other and more egregious naming abuses abound (see the table below, "The Water Comes from Where?"). "Arctic" is a hugely popular name for bottled water, symbolizing the legendary purity of the far frozen (albeit now rapidly melting) north, as are pictures and graphics of pristine frozen wildernesses or snow-covered mountain tops. Yet "Arctic Spring" water comes from Florida, while "Arctic Falls Bottled Water" and "Arctic Wolf Spring" brands come from

The Water Comes from Where?	
Bottled Water Label	**Water Source**
Arctic Wolf Spring	Philadelphia area, southern New Jersey
Arctic Clear	Bartlett, Tennessee
Arctic Falls Purified	Tulsa, Oklahoma
Arctic Falls Bottled	Cedar Grove, New Jersey
Arctic Springs	Los Angeles
Arctic Spring	Lakeland, Florida
Glacier Mountain Natural Spring	New Jersey
Glacier Mountain Bottled	Logan, Ohio
Glacier Bottled Water Company	Processed municipal water from vending machines
Glacier Spring	Victoria, Australia
Alaska Premium Glacier	Pipe 111241, Juneau Municipal Water*
Everest	Corpus Christi, Texas
Yosemite	Los Angeles municipal supply

* http://ezinearticles.com/?Water-Quality-of-Glaciers—Do-We-Want-It?&id=480313

New Jersey. "Arctic Falls Purified Water" is from Oklahoma and "Arctic Clear" from Tennessee. The consumer might reasonably expect that any bottled water with the name of Glacier would be lovingly collected by hand at the melt face of a pristine wilderness ice field, but no, sorry. "Glacier Mountain Natural Spring Water" is bottled in New Jersey. "Glacier Mountain Bottled Water" comes from Logan, Ohio, southeast of Columbus. The last time glaciers were seen in what is now New Jersey or Ohio was more than 10,000 years ago. The "Glacier Bottled Water" Company sells filtered municipal water from vending machines at grocery stores. Even "Alaska Premium Glacier" bottled water apparently came from the municipal water system in Juneau, "specifically, pipe # 111241."[10] At least it's really from Alaska, for whatever that's worth.

The FDA Standard Nutrition
Label for typical bottled water
showing, well, nothing.
[From www.nutritiondata.com.]

Nutrition Facts

Serving Size 1 fl oz 30g (29 g)
Servings per container 16

Amount Per Serving

Calories 0	Calories from Fat 0

	% Daily Value*
Total Fat 0g	0%
Saturated Fat 0g	0%
Trans Fat 0g	
Cholesterol 0mg	0%
Sodium 1mg	0%
Total Carbohydrate 0g	0%
Dietary Fiber 0g	0%
Sugars 0g	
Protein 0g	

Vitamin A	0%	• Vitamin C	0%
Calcium	0%	• Iron	0%

*Percent Daily Values are based on a 2,000 calorie diet.
Your daily values may be higher or lower depending on
your calorie needs:

	Calories	2,000	2,500
Total Fat	Less than	65g	80g
Sat Fat	Less than	20g	25g
Cholesterol	Less than	300mg	300mg
Sodium	Less than	2,400mg	2,400mg
Total Carbohydrate		300mg	375g
Fiber		35g	30g

Calories per gram:
Fat 9 • Carbohydrate 4 • Protein 4

©www.NutritionData.com

These kinds of misleading names aren't the exception—they seem to be the rule. "Yosemite" brand bottled water comes from the Los Angeles municipal water system. "Everest" brand water, complete with a picture of a tall snowy mountain on the bottle, comes from southeastern Texas, and while there are many big things in Texas, Mount Everest isn't one of them.

Don't expect regulators to step in and challenge these kinds of misrepresentations. Even with the FDA Standards of Identity, there are almost no requirements for truth in branding. Thus, a bottler can name a product "Glacier Bottled Water" but cannot call it "glacier water." Even the made-up names of Dasani and Aquafina are created by branding companies based on the responses of focus groups. When asked what the name "Dasani" means, Coca-Cola executives described consumer testing that "showed that the name is relaxing and suggests pureness and replenishment."[11] Is there any surprise consumers are easily fooled and misled?

So what is taking up all the space on the label? Other than graphic images of mountains or water or company logos, there is one more major component to a bottled water label in the United States—the standard FDA nutrition table. Because bottled water is considered a food product, the FDA requires bottlers to include the general "Nutrition Facts" food label on the bottle. We've all seen this standard label on food packages, which requires information be provided to the consumer on a range of things, from calories to fat content to vitamins. For real food, these labels can be useful. Not for water. Note the "information" on one such label that appears on a typical water bottle. No calories, no fat, no cholesterol, no sodium, no carbohydrates, no sugars, no protein, no vitamin A, no Vitamin C. Well, duh. None of these things are found in water. But there *are* things in water, lots of things. Even very clean and safe water has lots of dissolved minerals in it, and the composition of these minerals plays an important role in taste. By requiring bottled water in the United States to apply the standard food label, bottlers and regulators are misleading consumers about the safety, quality, and composition of that product, while at the same time failing to provide any useful information about what kinds of minerals are actually present. Compare the U.S. FDA label with the information typically presented on bottled waters in Europe, shown on page sixty-one.

More than a decade ago, the FDA concluded that it would be "feasible for the bottled water industry to provide the same type of information to consumers that the Safe Drinking Water Act requires" of public water systems, but they have taken no action to require the industry to do so, and apparently have no intention at present to do so.[12] There have been various attempts to strengthen and expand the kinds of information provided on water bottle labels, but these have almost always been beaten down by the industry. One recent example is California, which, in 2007, modestly tried to expand the information provided to consumers on water bottles, with bills from both the State Assembly and Senate. One provision of the Senate bill required that, as of January 1, 2009:

Each container of bottled water sold at retail or wholesale in this state in a beverage container shall include on its label, or on an additional label affixed to the bottle, or on a package insert or attachment, all the following:

(1) The name and contact information for the bottler or brand owner.

(2) The source of the bottled water, in compliance with applicable state and federal regulations.

(3) A clear and conspicuous statement that informs consumers about how to access water quality information. . . . [13]

The bill was supported by a broad coalition of consumer and community groups, public interest organizations, water utilities, and government agencies, including the Consumer Federation of California, the Association of California Water Agencies, the California League of Conservation Voters, Environment California, the Sierra Club, Environmental Defense, the Natural Resources Defense Council, Latino Issues Forum, the San Francisco Public Utilities Commission, and many more. Weak as it was, it was opposed by the California Bottled Water Association, California Chamber of Commerce, California Grocers Association, and the International Bottled Water Association. Why? The IBWA argued that "there has been no consumer demand for such measures," despite the fact that consumer groups strongly supported the California bills.[14] Some bottlers and representatives of the FDA tried to argue that there is not enough room on the label for this information, or that it would be too complicated or expensive to changes labels, even though some bottlers seem to find plenty of space and money to prepare fancy labels.[15] Nestlé Water North America actually has nine separate messages rotating through their bottled water labels, bragging about how environmental they are, how little plastic their eco-friendly bottles use, and so on.[16]

Mineral Constituents Typically Listed on European Mineral Water Labels*

1. Acidity (pH)
2. Total Dissolved Solids (TDS)
3. Aluminum (Al)
4. Arsenic (As)
5. Boron dioxide (BO2−)
6. Bromine (Br−)
7. Calcium (Ca++)
8. Chloride (Cl−)
9. Cobalt (Co)
10. Carbon dioxide (CO_2)
11. Chromium (Cr−)
12. Copper (Cu++)
13. Fluoride (F−)
14. Germanium (Ge)
15. Hardness
16. Hydrogen carbonate (HCO_3−)
17. Iodine (I)
18. Iron (Fe++)
19. Lithium (Li+)
20. Magnesium (Mg++)
21. Manganese (Mn+)
22. Nitrate (NO_3−)
23. Potassium (K+)
24. Rubidium (Rb)
25. Silica (SiO_2)
26. Sodium (Na+)
27. Strontium (Sr++)
28. Sulfate (SO_4−−)
29. Zinc (Zn++)

* http://www.mineralwaters.org/

The California legislature passed both bills, and Governor Schwarzenegger signed the Senate bill into law on October 13, 2007. While the new labels were supposed to be in place by January 2009, as of March 2009 many bottles of water on the shelves of my supermarket still lacked the new labels. Until better regulations on labeling are put in place, and are properly enforced, consumers will remain in the dark about what's really in the bottles of water we buy.

Ultimately, consumers should ask why bottled water is considered a "food" in the first place and whether it would make more sense to treat bottled water as, well, water, with the same rules, protections, and safeguards as tap water. A perfect example of the confusion generated by the FDA's regulations is the unusual case of "spring water." This class of bottled water dominates the U.S. market and consumers seem to prefer the cachet of spring water to processed municipal waters. But is it any better tasting or any safer? In order to answer this, we must first understand what spring water is and where it comes from.

CHAPTER 5

The Cachet of Spring Water

The mountain spring is the best.
— Kakuzo Okakura, *The Book of Tea*

High technology has done us one great service: It has retaught us the delight of performing simple and primordial tasks—chopping wood, building a fire, drawing water from a spring.
— Edward Abbey

ON A HOT summer day in 2007 I flew into the John Wayne International Airport in Burbank, California, rented a cheap compact car and headed east on Route 10, away from the smog and suburbia of Los Angeles toward the Mohave Desert and the Arizona state line. After months of negotiations, Nestlé Waters North America had finally given me permission to visit their Arrowhead Spring Water plant in Cabazon, California. Route 10 still rolls through patches of desert, but the expanses of open space are quickly being filled with identical versions of the same soulless suburban development that appears along the edges of every major highway in America.

Toward the town of Banning, the road is lined with evangelical billboards that advertise the coming Armageddon as though it were the latest Hollywood blockbuster, mixed with promotions for new cookie-cutter housing developments with names like Tournament Hills, Fairways, and Oak Valley, each with thirsty lawns and a golf course irrigated with water the desert can't afford to provide, taken from fossil groundwater aquifers that won't be recharged in our lifetimes.

A few dozen miles further east, just before you get to Palm Springs, lies the Morongo Indian Reservation near the desert town of Cabazon. This is a parched landscape, with sparse desert vegetation and winds that are so consistent and strong that companies are building massive wind farms here—vast forests of tall white turbine blades sweeping the air and converting the power of the wind into clean electricity.

Cabazon is an old stop on the Southern Pacific railroad line where the steam locomotives used to refill their boilers from a rare spring bubbling up from the side of Millard Canyon. The railroad built a rock-lined flume and ditch to bring the water down the wash to the rail line. When the roads killed the rails, the water was left to flow in its old channels, re-watering that rarest of ecosystems, the desert oasis.

Cabazon is still a major pit stop but now the attraction is the Morongo Indian casino and resort—a vast, ugly 27-story tower looming over the highway. I can see the casino from more than a dozen miles away and most drivers cannot resist the lure of the garish architecture, the discount chain stores in the mall, and the flashing neon lights promising a respite from miles of stark desert scenery. In fact, the casino so dominates the landscape that I completely missed my turnoff for one of the largest bottled water plants in the world—Nestlé's Cabazon Arrowhead Spring Water plant. I had to drive several more miles down the highway before I could turn around and try again. This is an incredibly incongruous place to find a bottled water plant. There just doesn't seem to be any water anywhere here in the heart of the Mohave Desert. But there is if you know where to look.

The Arrowhead plant is a low cavernous factory designed to blend into the landscape, and it looks like any other nondescript windowless industrial building, except that it covers an area larger than seven football fields. The outside landscaping is desert plants, though there is a small patch of nicely tended green lawn outside the employee lunchroom. Inside 220 employees produce more than 50 million cases—more than one billion bottles a year—of Arrowhead brand spring water. Outside, a nonstop stream of tractor-trailer trucks comes and goes, moving water in bulk or carrying finished product to stores.

It has taken me months and dozens of e-mails and phone calls to Nestlé's U.S. headquarters in Connecticut to get permission to visit. I'm met at the door by a group of Nestlé executives, including Heidi Paul, corporate vice president, and Nick Dege, director of quality assurance, both sent out from their Connecticut headquarters, as well as Kyle Kurst, the Cabazon plant director, and Larry Lawrence, the Cabazon plant's watershed-protection scientist. Dege literally wrote the book on the technology of bottled water, a copy of which sits on the reference shelf in my office.

In the 1970s Arrowhead was part of the Perrier Group of America and sold water from the original Arrowhead spring in the San Bernardino Mountains near Los Angeles to the home and office cooler market. In 1992 Nestlé bought the Perrier Group in a hostile takeover and started to expand operations to the individual plastic bottle market. As demand grew, Nestlé signed a contract with the Morongo Band of Mission Indians in Cabazon for access to their spring and built the Cabazon bottling plant, now one of Nestlé's flagships. The Cabazon facility was designed as one of the first bottling plants to meet the U.S. Green Building Council's LEED (Leadership in Energy and Environmental Design) standards for environmental sustainability. It also serves as a test platform for a number of Nestlé environmental initiatives, including lightweight bottles, wastewater recycling, and energy-efficiency efforts.

The real key to any bottled water plant is, of course, the water itself. In the case of the Cabazon plant, the water comes from a small desert spring a few miles away, hidden in the folds of Millard Canyon, upslope of the plant and the casino. The Banning earthquake fault line runs through the Canyon and forms an underground barrier that both defines one edge of a groundwater aquifer and offers a route for that water to reach the surface.

Water in the desert is a precious thing. In the western United States, every time water flows to the surface in the desert, an oasis appears—rare communities of life clustered around the precious resource of water. When water comes to the surface, it supports desert vegetation and even cottonwood trees, as well as beetles and other insects of remarkable design, spiders, fantastical solpugids that look like creatures from a horror movie on the SyFy channel, lizards, snakes, birds, and even rare fish. Sometimes these oases are temporary—ephemeral wetlands that ebb and flow with the availability of water. Brine shrimp and even some amphibians are capable of living in a state of suspended animation in dried earth in these ecosystems, reappearing with the rains for a brief period of frenzied eating and mating until the water disappears again.

But occasionally, here and there in small canyons and washes and protected pools, there is permanent water in the desert. These rare ecosystems are the most precious and vulnerable, because they depend on a delicate balance between inflow and outflow, gain and loss. Inflow is only rain, falling for short periods of time, in small amounts, which soaks into the groundwater table protected from evaporating in the hot sun. Where groundwater reaches the surface, it becomes a spring and a stream, flowing through the desert until either evaporation consumes it, it is taken up by plants and animals, or it seeps back down into the ground and disappears again.

If less water becomes available, whether because of a drop in rainfall or because humans start to extract it, there are only two possibilities: either groundwater levels drop or surface flows decrease. In the desert, both of these things happen until there is a new balance—a permanently lower level of groundwater and a permanent decrease in surface flows, which leads to a smaller oasis, a shorter desert stream, and an impoverished desert ecosystem.

The hydrologic cycle is actually pretty simple to understand: water comes in and goes out in various flows, and water sits around in various stocks and pools (both above and below the surface). Just like your bank account. When more water goes in than comes out, the amount of water stored goes up. When more water goes out than comes in, the water in storage goes down. Balance. Add a new demand like a bottled water plant and less water remains: either water levels drop or surface flows decrease. There is no alternative.

Much of the world's fresh water is stored as groundwater—water that seeps into soils over time from rainfall and accumulates in underground aquifers. Many people imagine that this water is in the form of vast pools, but groundwater is actually just saturated soil or rock layers that might be anywhere from a few feet to thousands of feet below the surface. A water well simply taps into these saturated layers and pumps water out. All groundwater originated as rainfall at one time or another—sometimes water pumped from wells can be just a few days old, sometimes it is literally tens of thousands of years old, laid down when the climate was wetter and stored safe from evaporating back into the atmosphere.

Water comes to the surface from underground aquifers through springs. There are many different kinds of springs. The simplest, like the Cabazon spring in Millard Canyon, flows when the level of groundwater is very close to the land surface and some kind of depression or landform permits the two to intersect. This is the case when springs issue from the side of a hill or at the bottom of a valley. Water from such springs is very closely connected to the land sur-face, and the water issuing from them typically fell very recently as rain. Often, such wells flow intermittently because the groundwater level rises and falls with natural rainfall.

Another kind of spring occurs when permeable sands or stone layers overlay an impermeable layer of clay or rock. The permeable layers fill up with water that seeps into the ground from rainfall or snowmelt and the water then moves sideways until it finds an outlet at the surface forming a spring. The waters in these kinds of ground-water basins are also typically relatively young and can be closely connected to the surface.

Under a few geological circumstances, rainwater can seep into the ground and percolate along faults and fractures into deep underground layers, where it may rest for centuries or millennia before returning to the surface along other faults where the level of the aquifer is higher than the outlet at the land surface. In these instances, or if a well is drilled into the formation, water will flow naturally from the spring or well. This is the definition of an artesian spring or well, and natural artesian wells are relatively rare. Such waters are less likely to be contaminated by animal or human wastes, or by industrial discharges, though they are more likely to have reacted chemically with the rocks around them and to contain higher levels of minerals.

A final kind of groundwater is deep fossil groundwater, where underground formations of permeable rock collect rainwater over long periods of time and store it, but where no surface outlets occur. Deep groundwater exists throughout the world and is increasingly being tapped for water supplies. While this water can often be very pure—indeed, in some places it was laid down thousands of years ago, long before the possibility of human or industrial contamination—its use is ultimately unsustainable if we tap into it and pump it at a faster rate than it is naturally recharged—just like oil. In many hot and arid regions of the world, deep groundwater aquifers have been discovered containing vast quantities of this "fossil" water, and some efforts have been made to tap them.

In North Africa, one of the hottest and driest regions of the world, such water supplies have been found under southern Libya, Chad, and Egypt. A decade ago Libyan leader Muammar Al Qadhafi launched a massive $30-billion project to drill wells and build a 5,000-kilometer-long pipeline to bring water from deep in the desert to the parched, arid coastal cities. Because this water is "fossil" water, pumping it is like pumping oil—the amount of water used is far higher than the rate of replenishment in the desert climate. Inexorably, the water level underground will fall, production will peak, and it will become too hard or costly to pump.

As Leonard Konikow, a hydrogeologist from the U.S. Geological Survey, told me at a UN-sponsored meeting in December 2008, any increase in withdrawal of groundwater must ultimately lead to a reduction in the amount of water stored in a basin or to a reduction in flow from surface streams connected to that groundwater. Pumping groundwater inevitably causes changes in nearby surface waters in cases where the two are connected. Robert Glennon succinctly puts it in his book *Water Follies*, "In fact, there is no sharp, meaningful distinction between surface and groundwater."[1] When groundwater rises to the level of the surface, we find springs and wetlands, and see water flows in local streams even when there has been no recent rain.

The close connection between many surface and groundwater systems raises two problems when we want to make use of water. The first is the possibility that groundwater pumping will affect the local watershed. The second problem is that contamination on the surface can lead to contamination of groundwater, especially "spring water" used for bottling. Pumping groundwater faster than nature recharges it can lower groundwater levels in local wells, dry up springs and streams, and destroy natural wetlands, even if substantial water remains underground. In a watershed with lots of rainfall and large flows, groundwater contributions are often only a small part of total runoff, and pumping groundwater may have little appreciable effect on surface flows. In a watershed where human use exceeds natural recharge, withdrawals of water inexorably decrease the level of groundwater.

We see this in the famous Ogallala aquifer under the Great Plains, in northern China, in parts of India, and elsewhere. The Ogallala contains ancient water slowly accumulated and stored over millennia. In recent decades, however, the Ogallala's modest inflows have been overwhelmed by massive agricultural pumping, and groundwater levels have dropped tens and even hundreds of feet. In some places, groundwater levels have fallen so far it is no longer economical for farmers to run their groundwater pumps, and they have reverted to dryland farming, while prairie potholes and surface springs have disappeared entirely. Despite these problems, some water companies still focus their efforts on bottling spring water because they believe their customers prefer it.

In the desert, it is especially easy to disturb the balance between inflow and outflow, and I'm interested to see how Nestlé will explain the implications of their plant on the Millard Canyon oasis. Lawrence leads us up to the site where Nestlé has drilled wells to tap the springs. Almost as if on cue, an immature red-tailed hawk bolts from a large cottonwood by the edge of the stream, which is barely but perceptibly flowing. This is sacred Indian ground, despite the fact that the Morongo Band of Mission Indians has leased the water to Nestlé and permitted wells to be dug to tap the spring. Hidden among the cottonwoods are artifacts like Indian grinding rocks. I can visualize a time when this precious desert stream was the center of a Native American community dependent on its perennial, reliable presence.

Nestlé argues that their plant has imposed no new impact on the canyon. This is quite possible if the previous water-rights holder was simply using the same amount of water for another purpose. A hundred years ago, small amounts of water were taken from this canyon to supply the steam engines of the Southern Pacific railroad on their way to and from the West Coast. But it is also true that the use of this water, for any purpose, is depriving the rare desert oasis of that same amount of water. If Nestlé were to stop pumping the 200 million gallons a year that they now extract, one of two things would happen: either the groundwater level would increase or the volume of water in the desert stream that flows down Millard Canyon would grow and the stream would flow much farther down the canyon before disappearing back into the ground or being absorbed by new vegetation and habitat. In all likelihood, both things would happen. Cottonwoods and other desert plants would reestablish themselves over a larger area, more precious habitat would be created, and insects, birds, amphibians, and lizards would return. There is, of course, an easy way to test this. Shut down the bottled water plant for a few weeks or months, and watch the groundwater levels rise or the flows in the stream grow. Nestlé is unlikely to conduct this test voluntarily, and no government agency seems likely to require it.

After being pumped to the surface, water flows through a pipe downhill to the Cabazon plant, where it undergoes additional processing, including microfiltration and treatment with ultraviolet light. This kind of processing filters out large particles and kills bacteria that might be in the water, but does not substantially alter the mineral content. The water is then pumped into 60,000-gallon silos before being bottled.

One of the first things I notice about the plant is how clean it is, inside and out. The place is so clean that I'd have no qualms about eating my sandwich off the floor, though of course I can't actually bring food into the plant. To enter the bottling facility itself, I have to don a plastic cap, paper booties, and a mask to cover my beard and moustache. Kyle Kurst, the plant director, walks us through the production lines. On the floor of the factory, massive Husky manufacturing machines are taking tiny little pellets of polyethylene terephthalate (PET) resin and making preforms, the precursors to the plastic bottles—thousands of them every minute.

These preforms are inspected and passed on to the state-of-the-art stretch/blowers, which heat them to 115 degrees C, stretch them, and blow them into the final familiar Nestlé bottle shape, ready for filling. Another machine grabs the newly formed bottles and races them through the filling stations, drawing treated water from the silos, capping the bottles, and testing them for fill level and a good seal. Bottles that leak or are not filled to the correct level are automatically plucked from the line and destroyed. Glue is applied to the properly filled bottles, followed by the label. A laser printer sprays batch numbers on the bottles, which are combined into case batches of 24, placed on corrugate, shrink wrapped, sprayed with an expiration date stamp, placed on pallets, and moved to the adjacent storage area packed floor to ceiling with completed pallets ready to be loaded onto trucks for delivery throughout the western United States. It is a remarkable dance of mechanical efficiency. The machines at Cabazon produce twenty-five hundred bottles a minute, a hundred and fifty thousand bottles an hour, three and a half million bottles a day. And similar operations around the country produce billions of gallons of spring water each year for dozens of other companies.

More than half of the bottled water sold in the U.S. comes from groundwater or from springs and is labeled "spring water." In order be able to use the term, the FDA requires a bottler to collect water directly from a spring or from a groundwater well that is hydrologically connected to a spring, and it cannot be processed or treated in any way that substantially changes its chemical composition. Many people prefer to buy spring water because it would seem to be natural, unprocessed, and protected from the kinds of contamination that may affect surface water, such as sewage, industrial discharges, animal wastes, and urban runoff. But is spring water really any better than other, more processed bottled waters? And what about the springs themselves?

Because so much bottled water comes from springs or groundwater wells, more and more communities with large bottling plants worry that their local wells, wetlands, and streams will be affected by large-scale commercial withdrawals. Part of the recent campaign against bottled water comes from such community concerns, and the industry has been working hard to address and discredit such worries as unfounded. In the face of growing concern over the local impact of water withdrawals by bottlers, the industry has conjured up misleading "science" to counter local opposition to proposed new bottling plants.

In 2004 the bottled water industry commissioned a research paper to show how insignificant their impact on groundwater was. This paper, funded by the Drinking Water Research Foundation, concluded that "relative to other uses of ground water, bottled water production was found to be a *deminimis* user of ground water. . . . Ground water withdrawals for bottled water production represent only 0.019% of the total fresh ground water withdrawals in the U.S."[2]

The DWRF is the "research" arm of the bottled water industry's lobby association. They share offices and staff with the bottled water industry group, the International Bottled Water Association (IBWA), which was quick to use these findings to counter growing political and legislative efforts against bottled water. "There is no scientific evidence of the bottled water industry's misuse or depletion of the Nation's renewable groundwater resources. In fact, bottled water accounts for less than 2/100's of a percent of all groundwater withdrawals in the United States."[3] Even the Australasian Bottled Water Institute and the Competitive Enterprise Institute, in their "Enjoy Bottled Water" campaign, latched onto this argument, citing the same industry paper.[4]

This conclusion is completely specious—so inappropriate on its face that the research article failed to pass peer review for scientific publication and has never appeared in a research journal. First, it argues against a hypothetical straw man: No opponent of bottled water has ever claimed that the industry is "deplet[ing] the Nation's renewable groundwater resources." Second, it uses an inappropriate and misleading comparison: What matters, of course, is not the total amount of groundwater used by the bottled water industry compared to total U.S. (or Australian, or New Zealand) use of groundwater. This kind of comparison would only make sense if all groundwater was one big, interconnected pool. It isn't. The comparison is akin to saying that the pollution from the stack of a dirty coal plant isn't a problem because the amount of air contaminated is a tiny fraction of all of the air over the entire United States. Tell that to the people who live in the neighborhood. What matters for air and for water, of course, is the effect on local communities.

What communities must worry about are the consequences of

bottled water production in the watershed where the plant is located. Should Californians worry about the effect of the Nestlé plant in Cabazon on the state's total groundwater supply? Of course not. Should someone worry about, monitor, and evaluate local groundwater impacts in Millard Canyon? Of course. When a bottled water plant is taking only a small part of the flows in a watershed, the impact can be modest, or even barely noticeable. But if a bottled water plant takes a significant fraction of the flows of water in a watershed, the impact can be large. And the impact is never *zero*. Yet bottlers are rarely asked, and even more rarely do they volunteer, to evaluate their impact in a detailed, analytical, scientifically defensible way.

These local realities, however, have not stopped the industry from posting the DWRF paper on its websites and citing the conclusions over and over again, in every forum where concern about groundwater withdrawals is raised. The paper has even been used by corporate lobbyists to oppose state regulation of bottled water withdrawals. In Michigan in 2007, for example, the Absopure bottled water company submitted the DWRF paper as part of its testimony before the Michigan House of Representatives, quoted the groundwater conclusion in their presentation, and made the grossly misleading and inappropriate argument that "bottled water appears to have no effect on water levels in the Great Lakes Basin as a whole."[5]

If the bottled water industry is misleading in its denial that groundwater withdrawals are a national problem, are bottled water opponents correct in accusing the industry of adversely affecting local water systems? Not always. In some places, bottled water plants use only a tiny fraction of the renewable water available in a region, and such a use of water needn't be a concern. But in other places, when detailed tests and studies are done, adverse impacts have indeed been found. In 2004 a bottled water plant planned for the Barrington, New Hampshire, region close to the border with Maine was opposed by local residents because of fear that the plant would cause local wells to dry up and wetlands to be destroyed. The company, USA Springs from Pelham, New Hampshire, wanted to build a bottling plant to pump over 300,000 gallons of water a day from an aquifer that underlies Nottingham, Barrington, and other towns in three watersheds. That amount would fill one million 20-ounce bottles every 24 hours. While it is entirely possible that pumping this volume of water would have only negligible effects upon local watersheds, the only way to find out is to actually test the effects. When the local officials required such a test over a ten-day period, portions of a critical local wetland dried up.[6]

In Maricopa County, Arizona, the Sedona Springs Bottled Water Company, operating under a permit granted by the Tonto National Forest, pumped enough groundwater to dramatically alter surface flows in Seven Springs Wash and the Spur Cross Ranch Conservation Area. The reduction in surface water led to the death of native fish, loss of leopard frogs and Mexican black hawks, the death of sycamore and ash trees, and die-back of deer grass. In July 2005 the company filed bankruptcy but continued to operate while it restructured, despite requests from the county to stop production.[7]

In Michigan, local activists took Nestlé Waters North America to court over plans to extract water from Sanctuary Springs, Michigan, for a large bottled water plant. The Michigan Court of Appeals in 2005 ruled that the use of groundwater for bottling is a beneficial use, providing employment and water to the general public. But they also found that the level of pumping proposed by Nestlé "would be unreasonable" and would adversely affect another reasonable use—the recreational, aesthetic, and environmental values of surface streams connected to the groundwater—by cutting flows, raising water temperatures, and reducing habitat. The court thus explicitly required an evaluation of the connections between surface and groundwater, as well as an assessment of a reasonable rate of water extraction that would balance environmental, social, and commercial interests.[8] Shouldn't this kind of evaluation be standard?

Even when pumping groundwater and bottling spring water has a noticeable effect on local water resources, some bottlers argue that spring water is more natural than processed waters. But does this

mean it is any safer? On the contrary, there are reasons to be especially concerned about the safety of spring waters precisely because
they receive less treatment than reprocessed municipal waters.
Municipal water, after all, is already considered safe to drink under
the EPA's regulations. And as for spring water, there are loopholes
in U.S. regulations that open the door to contamination by viruses
and other pathogenic organisms, such as *Cryptosporidium, Legionella,*
and *Giardia lamblia.*

This class of organisms is increasingly found in surface water
and has also been found in groundwater. We learned the hard way
about the dangers of these pathogens in drinking water. *Cryptosporid-*
ium in Milwaukee's municipal water was implicated in a severe
water-related disease outbreak in 1993 that killed one hundred people and sickened hundreds of thousands more. That outbreak lead to
stricter tap water filtration rules nationwide. Yet the FDA has
refused to establish a bottled water regulation for these organisms.
Why? The bottled water lobby argues, and the FDA so far agrees,
that because bottled water largely comes from one of two general
sources, municipal water and spring water, it is protected. Municipal
water is now required by the EPA to be free of these organisms
under federal drinking water regulations. "Spring" water is simply
defined by the FDA as free from the influence of surface water and
thus *assumed* to be free from these organisms. No federal tests are
required to confirm the lack of "direct influence," and no clear definition of "direct influence" is applied. Like the FDA argument about
the absence of certain bacteria (i.e., there's no need to regulate for
them or inspect for them, because they are not *supposed* to be in bottled water), this is classic circular reasoning: bottlers don't need to
test for these contaminants because regulators simply assume
they're not in the water.

In addition to being circular reasoning, it is simply wrong. As
I've noted above, almost all groundwater originates at some point as
surface water and there are often close physical connections, expos-
ing groundwater to surface water contamination. According to the

EPA, approximately 27 percent of groundwater wells studied some-times have viral contamination.9 As a result, the EPA recently con-cluded that existing regulations for groundwater systems fail to adequately address the risk of groundwater contamination from surface sources, and they fail to adequately require monitoring or disinfection of contaminated groundwater when it is discovered. According to the agency's own report, "EPA determined that there is the potential for ground water to be contaminated with pathogenic bacteria or viruses, or both, and that the presence of fecal indicators can demonstrate a pathway for pathogenic enteric bacteria or viruses to enter GWSs [ground water sources]."10

As a result of this finding, the EPA now explicitly requires tap water that comes from groundwater to be tested to determine if these contaminants exist, and it requires municipal water to be treat-ed to ensure these contaminants are removed. The same require-ment doesn't exist for bottled water.

In fact, groundwater sources are often found, when actually test-ed, to be both at risk of contamination or actually contaminated. An outbreak of cryptosporidiosis in North London in March 1997 was traced to a contaminated groundwater supply, and the Drinking Water Inspectorate of the United Kingdom Department of the Envi-ronment, Transport, and Regions reported that "Evidence is accu-mulating worldwide for the potential for contamination of groundwater by *Cryptosporidium*." As the British scientists conclud-ed: "Not all groundwater is consistently high quality." They went on to recommend that water utilities "should be especially vigilant for the possibility of intermittent rapid transmission of water from the surface into boreholes, wells, and springs. The catchment, resource, and source characteristics should always be reviewed against water quality data. If it is necessary to undertake further work, sampling should include recharge periods or times when . . . surface water are most contaminated."11

Studies in Italy, Brazil, and the U.S. have all found the same thing: *Cryptosporidium* in groundwater wells thought to be protected from contamination.[12] An Italian study found these contaminants in deep groundwater wells. A Brazilian study found *Cryptosporidium* oocysts in groundwater used for human consumption in Itaquaquece-tuba City in Sao Paulo, Brazil.[13] In the United States scientists took samples from 199 vertical and horizontal wells and springs in 23 states and tested them for *Cryptosporidium* and *Giardia*. Twelve percent of the sites were positive for at least one of the contaminants, with greater contamination at springs than vertical wells. In particular, the scientists found *Cryptosporidium* oocysts in 5 percent of the vertical wells, 20 percent of the springs, 50 percent of the infiltration galleries, and 45 percent of the horizontal wells.[14] A follow-on study from 166 sites found similar contamination and concluded that the only way to determine if groundwater and springs in the United States are truly free of contamination is to test them.[15] Until bottlers are required to do these tests, we will remain in the dark about what's really in the bottles of spring water we buy and consumers will be at risk.

Nestlé's massive Cabazon plant is a model of efficiency, cleanliness, and productivity. It helps Nestlé satisfy a growing demand for spring water in the western United States, and they (and their competitors) are seeking to build dozens more plants to tap into the nation's natural groundwater systems. But consumers should know that there is no guarantee that spring water is better or safer than any other water, and that it sometimes comes at a high cost to our natural ecosystems, hidden in our desert canyons and pristine wetlands.

CHAPTER 6

The Taste of Water

Eh. Water is water. It all tastes the same to me.
— Security guard standing next to the bottled water
  bar serving ten varieties of bottled water at the
  2006 International Bottled Water Association
  Convention in Los Angeles[1]

There's no accounting for taste.
— My mother

A FEW MONTHS after my visit to Nestlé's Cabazon plant, I turn into the parking lot of a factory in a nondescript industrial district alongside Route 880 between Oakland and San Jose. I'm here to visit Coca-Cola's San Leandro bottling plant, one of a thousand bottling plants associated with the world's largest beverage company. In the midst of production lines of Coke Classic, Diet Coke, Vanilla Coke, Coca-Cola Zero, Caffeine-Free Diet Coca-Cola, Cherry Coke, and other beverages are machines that take water from the city of San Leandro's municipal taps and convert it into Coca-Cola's flagship water product: Dasani.

The process in San Leandro is remarkably similar to the process used to produce spring water. As I walk through the plant, I'm shown where water comes into the factory, receives treatment, is put into bottles, and shipped out to local distributors. The machines and production lines look similar to Cabazon. The speed and efficiency are the same. There are really only a couple of differences. First, the source of water here is municipal tap water that has already been treated to meet federal standards. And second, because the product isn't going to be labeled "spring" water, Coca-Cola can put the water through more intensive purification systems. Indeed, Dasani is typically processed with combinations of state-of-the-art filtering, ultraviolet purification, ozonation, and reverse osmosis systems, which strip out almost all minerals. In fact, reverse osmosis removes so many minerals that the water doesn't taste good—some minerals are required for a decent taste. By necessity, therefore, Coca-Cola then adds a carefully prepared mix of minerals—"pixie dust" some in the industry call it—*back* into the water to create a finished product with a standardized taste, no matter where the water originated or was processed. Thus, Dasani from San Leandro is virtually indistinguishable from Dasani from Detroit, or New York, or any of the other local plants that produce it, even when the source waters taste quite different. Similarly, PepsiCo's Aquafina brand, Nestlé's Pure Life brand, and other bottlers that use reprocessed municipal sources all produce bottled waters that are almost indistinguishable from each other. This raises a new challenge for bottlers. How can people's taste buds be used to sell bottled water, if the taste differences are minor or non-existent?

You can never really tell who is going to like what, or why. People certainly have taste preferences, sometimes extremely subtle ones. And we're often willing to go out of our way to experience, or avoid experiencing, certain tastes. My mother would rarely, but occasionally, cook liver as a special treat for my father, who loved it, while the rest of the family practically had to eat in another room because it so grossed us out. Taste is a tongue-nose thing, scientists tell us. The tongue has millions of little chemical sensors, called papillae, capable of detecting and differentiating among different chemical compounds. The nose has its own set of sensors, called olfactory cells, that can distinguish among thousands of different odors. The combination of these detectors sends signals that the brain converts to taste and smell.

People tell me all the time, often apologetically, that the reason they buy bottled water is that they just don't like the taste of their tap water. But survey after survey has shown that few people can actually tell the difference among bottled waters or between bottled water and tap water when tasting water samples served out of identical unmarked containers at the same temperature. In May 2005 ABC News' 20/20 broadcast a report on a taste test in New York City where they offered five bottled waters and city tap water in a blind test. Even people who thought they didn't like the taste of NYC tap water often preferred tap water over costly bottled waters. And the most expensive water turned out to be the one people liked least. A 2008 taste test in London compared local tap water with more than two dozen brands of bottled water. London tap water came in third.[2] In October 2006, 80 percent of the 650 participants in a water taste test in Wandsworth, England, couldn't tell the difference between tap water and leading bottled water brands, and indeed, two-thirds of them preferred the taste of tap water to bottled water.[3]

These kinds of results no longer surprise me. I've participated in dozens of formal and informal water taste tests myself, and watched many more. Given a sample of three or four waters, I can often tell that they taste slightly different. But I can almost never tell which is which—bottled from tap, or brand A from brand B—and I rarely have a strong preference among them. And test after test shows the same things: people think they don't like tap water, but they do. Or they think they can distinguish the taste of their favorite bottled water, but they can't. Or the results of these tests are little different from random guessing. Just do a YouTube search for "bottled water taste test" and you'll have dozens of examples from which to choose.

We can certainly tell the differences between different kinds of wines or coffees—and a few people with consistent and discerning palates have made a very good living tasting things and selling their tastes to rest of us. We rely on these "experts" all the time to make decisions for us. Take wine for example. I know what I like when I taste it, but I've never been able to find an expert whose tastes reliably match mine so that I can stop randomly buying bottles of wine in the hopes of finding ones I like. Robert Parker, perhaps the most influential wine critic in the world, is the classic example of a taste "expert." His point system for wines produces numbers that can make or break vineyards and determine prices even when people have no idea if his taste preferences correspond to their own.

When I was growing up, I loved watching the Savarin coffee commercials showing the mythical El Exigente—"the demanding one." This iconic taste tester (played on TV by Carlos Montalbán, brother of actor Ricardo Montalbán) could single-handedly determine the future of poor coffee growers in Latin America by deciding whether their coffee tasted good enough to be purchased for Savarin. The commercials showed entire poor communities standing in the village square holding their collective breath waiting for El Exigente to taste the fruits of their labors and pass judgment on whether, presumably, the village would be able to sell their crop, feed and clothe their children, and survive until the next harvest. I always held my breath too, until he would put down the cup of coffee, smile, and nod his approval, leading to an instant and raucous celebration.

I doubt El Exigente would pass political muster today. That commercial, viewed through today's eyes, reveals some pretty remarkable facts about taste, global trade, poverty, and the power of international corporations. It shows how we regularly cede to others all sorts of decisions about taste. It reveals the power of a small number of people or corporations to make decisions that make or break the lives of many others. And it highlights how smart and effective advertising and marketing can often lead us to make consumer choices that are different from the ones we would make if we were doing our own tasting, whether of wine, coffee, music, politicians, or bottled water.

Different waters certainly can have different tastes. Bottled water can come from natural springs, rainwater, glacier melt, deep underground aquifers, desalinated ocean water, or municipal water supplies (which themselves come from many different sources), and it can be processed in dozens of different ways that alter its natural mineral content and taste. Early bottled water sellers capitalized on these differences, selling waters with varying concentrations of naturally occurring minerals and very different tastes. In the 1800s, both in the United States and Europe, the market was dominated by a small number of high-end bottlers producing medicinal waters, such as Poland Spring, Saratoga Springs, and a wider range of European mineral waters, such as Vichy, Marienbad, Vittel, Evian, Carlsbad, and Perrier. A book written by Dr. J. J. Moorman in 1873 on "Mineral Springs of North America" describes in detail dozens of springs and their supposed medicinal properties.[4] In 1899 another such comprehensive directory with hundreds of mineral water springs was written by Dr. James King Crook.[5] By 1905 a regular bulletin, "Mineral Waters of the United States," was being published by the U.S. Department of Agriculture, describing natural mineral waters throughout the United States. Even today, much of the bottled water industry in Europe is built around natural mineral waters. Europeans are much more likely to favor particular brands of sparkling or still mineral water because they like a particular taste. In the United States, however, the water market is now dominated by the blander, processed, low-mineral-content waters sold by the larger corporate beverage companies.

This partly explains the differences in labeling described earlier. The European tradition of expansive labels that provide a long list of minerals came about because those different minerals have different implications for taste, and people used to know what specific brands of bottled water they liked. In a sophisticated analysis of minerals and taste, Drs. Juyun Lim and Harry T. Lawless of Cornell University's Department of Food Science tested for taste sensations from salts of iron, calcium, magnesium, zinc, and other minerals commonly found in food and water.[6] Subjects were asked whether specific solutions and combinations of these minerals tasted sweet, sour, salty, metallic, bitter, or astringent. Sodium chloride salts tasted, well, salty to most participants. Alum tasted astringent to some and sour to others. Iron compounds were typically described as tasting metallic, but sometimes were also described as both sour and sweet. Calcium salts were often considered bitter, salty, or astringent. Magnesium salts were thought to be a combination of bitter, astringent, and metallic. Zinc was astringent. And so on. It should be no surprise, therefore, that the complex combinations of minerals in some waters lead to complex taste variations and perceptions.

A website devoted to mineral waters—www.mineralwaters.org —lists literally thousands of brands and their mineral compositions. Interested in a high-salt mineral water? Try Aachener Kaiserbrunnen, first bottled in 1884 in Bad Aachen, Germany, and containing nearly 1,300 milligrams per liter (mg/l) of sodium. You can't grow many crops using water with this much salt. In contrast, Arctic Ice (from Victoria, Australia, and containing neither ice nor any water from the Arctic) has less than 10 mg/l of sodium. Like your water with lots of sulfates and bicarbonate? Then try Fontechiara from Parma, Italy, with 111 mg/l and 354 mg/l of those minerals. In contrast, Dias D'Avila from Bahia, Brazil, lists only 2 mg/l of sulfates and less than 10 mg/l of bicarbonate.

Given the vast differences in the mineral content of different waters from different sources, it should come as no surprise that sooner or later, high-end restaurants would see an opportunity to take advantage of both the confusion about the taste of water and the profit opportunities in offering expensive bottled water. Enter "water sommeliers"—the water version of the wine experts at restaurants, only in this case they help diners match different waters with different foods while also boosting restaurant profits.

The first reported water sommelier was hired at the Ritz-Carlton in New York City in 2002, but by 2007 the press was full of news of restaurants from Toronto to Sydney to the major cities in Europe offering water menus and hiring people to help customers buy expensive bottled water.[7] In March 2007 Badoit, which supplies one of the sparkling waters served in many Parisian restaurants, started offering a course in "eaunologie" ("eau" means water in

French and "eaunologie" is a play on the French word *oenologie*, the science of wine).[8] These are being run by Dominique Laporte, the sommelier at the famed Alain Senderens restaurant. Laporte adopts the language of wine experts to describe bottled waters, talking about their "nose" and "ending," among other characteristics.[9] Peter Bell, the sommelier of Astral in Sydney, Australia, added a water menu of five still and five sparkling waters. "In Europe, having eight or nine waters on the menu is standard," said Bell.[10]

Perhaps the fanciest effort to promote bottled water in restaurants was the decision by Claridge's, the famous London Hotel on Brook Street, to offer a water menu featuring thirty different high-end water brands from around the world. Claridge's menu includes water from the Tai Tapu volcano in New Zealand, an Italian brand reportedly favored by the Pope, bottled rainwater from Australia, desalinated deep ocean water from Hawaii, and spring water from the Nilgiris Mountains in India. Each water is described in loving terms, such as "a pleasant smooth sensation on the palate," "slightly sweet taste and is the perfect accompaniment to sushi," and "distinctively soft taste goes well with salads." "Water is becoming like wine," Claridge's food and beverage director Renaud Grégoire told a reporter. "Every guest has an opinion and asks for a particular brand." Of course this water comes at a price. One brand is listed at £50 a liter and several more cost over £20 a liter. Fortunately, diners can still order free London tap water. A spokesman for London's water system noted, "Our water is of the highest standard and it costs less than a tenth of a penny per litre."[11]

The best-known water sommelier, however, doesn't actually exist. He is the creation of the magicians, humorists, and scientific debunkers Penn and Teller and can be found on YouTube. In their short-lived but cultishly popular cable TV series, "Bullshit!" Penn and Teller created a fictitious water bar at a popular upscale restaurant, complete with an actor playing a water sommelier armed with a printed menu of fancy bottled water choices, including "L'Eau de Robinet" (literally "tap water" in French), "Mt. Fiji" water, and others. The water steward lovingly describes the differences among the choices to customers: "its aggressive flavor and brash attitude make it a perfect complement to meats and poultry," and "known throughout the Far East for its clean and bracing flavor." As different waters are served, we watch a series of painfully embarrassing scenes of customers exclaiming enthusiastically over the clear and subtle differences in taste that they think they can discern among the different bottles, and how much better their expensive bottled water is than tap water. "Oh yeah, definitely better than tap water." "Very fresh taste to it." "Better than L.A. County water." "Smoother than tap water." Meanwhile, in the back of the restaurant we see the fancy bottles all being filled from the same garden hose with, as Penn and Teller put it, "premium hose water."

Some tap water really does taste bad. But the solution is not to give up and move to bottled water. Rather consumers must demand that water agencies adjust the chemical composition of tap water to a potable, and palatable, level. If most of us can't really taste the difference between bottled water and tap water, or even prefer tap water in blind taste tests, why do we buy so much bottled water? Part of the answer is convenience—it has become harder and harder to find a public water fountain anymore, even in high-traffic areas like schools and sports arenas. And conversely, the bottled water industry has done what it can to make their product as convenient and readily accessible as possible. Think about where you are right now: there may be no water fountain nearby, but you can probably find someone selling a plastic bottle filled with water within a few hundred feet.

CHAPTER 7

The Hidden Cost of Convenience

We are a 24/7 on-the-go society who wants convenience in our beverage choices.
— Kim E. Jeffery, CEO, Nestlé Waters North
   America, May 21, 2008

There is no reason that the universe should be designed for our convenience.
— John D. Barrow, English physicist and mathematician

Mr. McGuire: I want to say one word to you. Just one word.
Benjamin: Yes, sir.
Mr. McGuire: Are you listening?
Benjamin: Yes, I am.
Mr. McGuire: Plastics.
— From the film *The Graduate* (1967)

"WE, John Rex Whinfield, of Meyroyd, Hollins Lane, Accrington, in the County of Lancaster, and James Tennant Dickson, of 26, Ormingston Crescent, East Lothian, Scotland, both British Subjects, do hereby declare the nature of this invention to be as follows . . ."

These words announced the discovery and patenting of the material that would eventually become the key to the explosive growth of the sales of bottled water—the plastic throwaway bottle. If the only containers available for water were glass or aluminum cans, I believe that sales of bottled water would never have taken off.

In 1941, forty-year-old John Rex Whinfield was employed as a research chemist by the Calico Printer's Association, a small English fabric company. Whinfield's job focused on the chemistry of fabric dyeing and finishing for the war effort, but in his spare time, he studied the molecular makeup and properties of synthetic fibers. In March of that year, Whinfield and his 21-year-old assistant, James Dickson, discovered a method of condensing terephthalic acid and ethylene glycol to produce a magical new material that could be drawn into fibers with a high melting point and a strong resistance to biodegradation. This material became known as "polyethylene terephthalate" (PET or PETE), or polyester, or Dacron, and after World War II it rapidly became the most widely produced synthetic fiber in the world. It surpasses nylon in both toughness and resilience and it can be made into any number of forms, including fabrics, rugs, strapping material, films, recording tape, mylar, and especially, lots and lots of plastic bottles.

Portability has always been a problem for water. Simply put, water is remarkably heavy. One gallon weighs eight pounds. A cubic meter of water—imagine a cube about three feet by three feet by three feet—literally weighs a ton. The picturesque images we see of women in Africa carrying water on their heads from a village well or stream belie a backbreaking and grueling chore. Try it yourself: Fill a plastic container with four or five gallons of water and carry it around the block.

The earliest water containers were probably simple hollowed gourds or the bladders of large animals. Archeologists have also come upon early water containers made of earthenware, fired and glazed pottery, and stone. One of the most famous references to stone water containers appears in the Gospel of St. John:

> And there were set there six waterpots of stone, after the manner of the purifying of the Jews, each containing two or three firkins apiece (John 2:6).
> And Jesus saith unto them, Fill the water pots with water. And they filled them up to the brim (John 2:7).[1]

Recycling Codes for Plastics

There are many kinds of plastics and in 1988 the Society of the Plastics Industry introduced a classification scheme to help consumers identify different forms and to aid recycling efforts. This resulted in the triangular symbols that are embossed on most plastic items and increasingly familiar to consumers.

PETE

polyethylene terephthalate — e.g., water bottles and soda bottles

HDPE

high density polyethylene — e.g., Tupperware; milk jugs, plastic bags, auto gas tanks

V

vinyl/poly vinyl chloride — e.g., window cleaners, vinyl siding, pipes.

LDPE

low density polyethylene — e.g., squeezeable mustard, those annoyingly useful six-pack soda can rings, plastic bags.

PP

polypropylene — e.g., yogurt containers, the lid of your Tic-Tac box, warm weather clothing, rope.

PS

polystyrene — e.g., egg cartons, those horrible foam drink cups, and common packing materials.

OTHER

"other" plastics, including polycarbonate (Lexan), plastics made of mixed resins or multiple layers

As the technology of containers improved, stone, clay, and ceramics gave way to wooden barrels and glass. In the nineteenth century, glass bottles were commercially produced and used for bottling mineral waters. Even today, many higher-end mineral waters come exclusively in glass bottles and collectors seek out old versions of water bottles at auctions and antique stores, and on eBay. But even for expensive bottled water, sales in glass are limited. Glass is heavy, which adds to the cost of producing and shipping it, and it breaks easily. After the Korean War, the widespread availability of aluminum led to the development of the aluminum can to replace

Is Water from Plastic Bottles Safe?

Part of the opposition to bottled water comes from concerns over the safety of the plastics used for packaging and whether these plastics leach dangerous chemicals into the product we drink. It should be no surprise that consumers are confused about the safety and environmental consequences of plastics and the chemicals used to make them. Who can blame us? Our society has shown a remarkable ability to create new weird chemical mixtures and combinations of materials. And industry has been able to get them into commercial production in massive quantities far faster than our scientists and regulatory agencies have been able to test them for their environmental and human health consequences.

History is rife with examples of smart things we did with magical new materials that turned out to be stupid. DDT—that wonderful pesticide that kills more than pests. MTBE—the gasoline additive that solves an air pollution problem while causing a far more serious water pollution problem. Dioxin—a byproduct of dozens of industrial activities and superb at causing cancer and reproductive failures. CFCs—stable chemicals that are effective for air conditioning and firefighting and, alas, also remarkably effective at destroying the Earth's ozone layer. Perc (or perchloroethylene)—fantastic for dry cleaning and also for causing dizziness, fatigue, headaches, unconsciousness, irritation of skin, eyes, nose, and throat, liver and kidney damage, memory loss, confusion, and, oh yes, cancer.

We already know that some plastics should not be used for water or food. Polyvinyl chloride (PVC) leaches phthalates, a hormone disruptor, and dioxin, a carcinogen. Polystyrene can leach styrene, a possible human

continued

individual steel and tin food containers, though all-aluminum cans were not used for carbonated soft drinks until the early 1960s. Aluminum cans then rapidly dominated the beverage market because of their convenience, light weight, and recyclability. Aluminum containers, however, are not commonly used for water because they impart a slight taste to their contents. When the contents are soft drinks or fruit juices, this taste is effectively undetectable. When the content is water, the taste is far more apparent.

Enter plastics, specifically Whinfield and Dickson's invention "polyethylene terephthalate" or PET. PET is easily recognized by the resin identification number 1, as illustrated on p. 89. This particular form of plastic has some wonderful characteristics of special

Is Water from Plastic Bottles Safe?, *continued*

carcinogen. But what about the PET or polycarbonate commonly used for bottled water? PET is widely considered to be one of the safest forms of plastic for food packaging, and few credible studies have ever claimed to find a risk of leaching.

Not so for some other materials: some bottled water, especially bottled water sold in large sizes for office or home coolers, is packaged in polycarbonate (PC), which is stronger than PET for large volumes of water. Lexan water bottles are also made of polycarbonate. Under some extreme conditions, such as the cleaning of polycarbonate with abrasive materials, or long-term storage of water in PC containers, some PC appears to release bisphenol A (BPA), a potentially serious health hazard. A contentious and active debate in the health community is underway about both the extent of leaching and the human health implications of exposure to BPA. I have no doubt that we'll learn more in the coming years as the science improves, and I urge more research on leaching risks and health consequences of all plastics used for water or food.

What should a wary consumer do in the meantime? I certainly wouldn't drink water that has sat around in a hot car in any kind of plastic bottle for several days. Even if the plastic doesn't leach, heat and light encourage bacterial growth. Cautious consumers can now find newer polycarbonate bottles made without BPA or buy lightweight stainless steel or enamel-lined aluminum bottles. And finally, tap water is so cheap that you can afford to empty your reusable bottle and refill it with clean fresh water as often as you like.

---

interest to the food and beverage industry. It is resistant to heat, mineral oils, solvents, and acids. It is impermeable to carbonation. It is strong, light, impact resistant, naturally transparent, and completely recyclable. And it doesn't impart a taste to its contents. As a result, PET is the most common plastic used for food packaging. The research available today also suggests that PET does not leach chemicals into the water, unlike many other types of plastic.

PET entered the commercial soft drink market in 1977, but bottled water in PET didn't appear until 1990, when Nestlé introduced the plastic water bottle.[2] "It revolutionized our industry," said Kim Jeffrey, CEO of Nestlé Waters North America, "because now people could get bottled water in the same format they were getting soft drinks in." Today the vast majority of bottled water sold in the United States—more than 95 percent—is packaged in PET containers.3 If you get your bottled water in large five- or six-gallon jugs that sit on top of a cooler, you are probably getting water packaged in polycarbonate (PC), not PET. Polycarbonate has greater strength in larger volumes, but research suggests it can leach bad chemicals into the water.

I love the TV show *How It's Made*, produced in Quebec, Canada. I can sit happily for thirty minutes and watch how factories, smart machines, and skilled workers make baseball bats, kayaks, bicycle safety helmets, or gumball machines. And for bottled water, the process is equally fascinating. Almost all PET bottles are produced through stretch/blow molding. The first step involves making pure PET "resin" in the form of pellets resembling grains of rice. This resin is the raw material used to make a wide range of different PET products. In the United States in 2008, total PET resin consumption was about 4 million tons, with domestic production coming from seven main producers: Starpet, Eastman, Nan Ya Plastics, M&G Polymers, Dak Americas, Wellman, and Invista.4 Around a million tons of this product goes to the bottled water industry.

To make beverage bottles, resin is injected into heated forms that mold it into "preforms." A preform looks like a thick-walled test tube with the same weight as the final bottle and with a finished neck and set of cap threads (or as several different industry salesmen told me at a trade show, "a very small hard condom with a screw cap"). Preforms are then heated, stretched, and blown into the final bottle shape in machines that can make literally hundreds of bottles a minute. Some major bottlers do the whole thing: take resin, make preforms, and blow, fill, and package their own bottles. Most smaller bottlers buy bottles that were blown somewhere else and then fill them in a bottling plant. When I toured the massive Nestlé Arrowhead plant in Cabazon, California, I was transfixed by the machines gobbling up tiny little round pellets of pure plastic resin and spitting out hundreds of bottles a minute, automatically testing them for

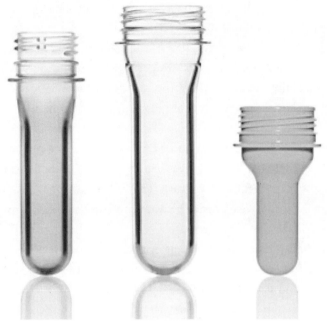

PET preforms. From http://www.pdg-plastiques.com/Portals/0/preformes.jpg

flaws, rejecting bad ones, and sending good ones zipping off to the next set of machines to be filled with water, capped, labeled, and packaged. From start to finish, the entire process of turning raw plastic into a finished bottle of water ready to be shipped to a store takes only a few minutes. At a modern bottled water plant, millions of throwaway PET bottles can be produced each day.

This convenience comes at a cost. As we become increasingly savvy consumers and learn more about the implications of our purchases for natural resources and the environment, new and complicated questions arise. Were those inexpensive running shoes made by child labor in bad working conditions? Was the cotton in my blue jeans grown organically and with efficient irrigation? Are the Central American coffee growers who provided the beans for my morning cup being fairly compensated? What is the carbon footprint of my daily commute? And what are the true costs of my convenient plastic water bottle—the costs of making the plastic bottle and shipping it to me as well as the environmental costs of disposing of the plastic garbage when I'm done drinking?

Resources are required to make, package, transport, chill, use, and recycle bottled water and its packaging, including both energy and, ironically, water. Making the plastic for a liter bottle of water actually takes three or four more liters of water itself. The real problem, though, is the energy cost: PET itself is typically made from petroleum. Making a kilogram of PET, which is enough for around 30 one-liter plastic bottles, takes around 3 liters of petroleum. More energy is then required to turn that PET into bottles, to filter, ozonate, or otherwise purify the water, to run the bottling machines, and to chill the bottle before use.

And even more substantively, it takes a lot of energy—almost all in the form of fossil fuels—to move the finished product to the place where you buy it. The total transportation energy requirement depends on two major factors: the distance and the mode of transportation. Unlike purified water from municipal sources, which are typically bottled and sold locally, "spring" waters must be packaged at specific sources and transported, sometimes significant distances. As we've seen, Nestlé bottles water under the Arrowhead label at several plants in Southern California for distribution throughout their western markets, and the company bottles water under the Poland Spring label in Maine for distribution throughout the eastern United States. This water usually travels in trucks, which take more energy to move the same kilogram of stuff than do trains or cargo ships. Even more extreme examples include the specialty waters that travel overseas, like Fiji Natural Artesian water, which is packaged at its source in the South Pacific, or Evian water, which is packaged at its source in France, and then shipped to markets around the world.

The transportation energy cost thus varies significantly, depending on our choices as consumers. If you live in L.A. and buy Fiji Water, the energy cost of transporting the water to you is equal to the energy embodied in the plastic bottle itself. If you live in L.A.

and can't do without Evian from France, the transportation energy involved is even higher. If you can't do without Fiji on your private jet, the most energy-intensive form of transport—well, you're probably not thinking much about your energy costs anyway. Put all of these different pieces together—materials, production, and transportation—and the energy costs of bottled water can be the oil equivalent of a quarter or more of the volume of the bottle. And this energy cost is a thousand times larger than the energy required to procure, process, treat, and deliver tap water. A study I conducted with my colleague Heather Cooley and published in *Environmental Research Letters* in 2009 concluded that global production and use of bottled water required the equivalent of between 100 and 160 million barrels of oil in 2007, along with all of the concomitant environmental consequences of getting and using fossil fuels.5

What about the environmental consequences of the bottles when we're done with them? How can we deal with the huge volumes of plastic waste that bottled water use generates? If bottled water isn't going to disappear, what can we do to reduce the environmental consequences of this waste? Obviously, the first thought of many is simply to stop buying the bottles. But short of this solution, unlikely in the near term, there are five possibilities for our empty bottles: Throw them away, recycle them, reduce the amount of packaging used for each bottle, burn them for energy, or make the bottles out of something else entirely that may have less environmental impact.

At least three-quarters of our water bottles are thrown out and end up in one of the nation's landfills—or lying in the gutter at the side of the road. Even if the bottled water consumer is responsible enough to throw the empty bottle in the garbage, rather than just on the ground, the path to the landfill is depressingly short and the consequences effectively permanent. PET doesn't degrade or compost. I live in a small single-family house in Berkeley, California. If I fail to recycle and put a used plastic water bottle in my regular gray garbage can, it is picked up at my curb on Thursday morning by a local city garbage truck. When that truck is full, it heads off to the City of

Berkeley transfer facility down near the highway, where it dumps its load. Very few cities around the world make any effort to recover recyclable materials from the general waste stream—it is hard to do and expensive, often requiring either poorly performing automated separation machines, or poorly paid hand labor. In Berkeley, as in cities all over the world, the day's collected garbage is compacted without being sorted for recoverable materials and then loaded into larger trucks that take it out to one of two local landfills, where, by the end of the day, that plastic bottle will join tons of other waste for centuries to come. I have this recurring fantasy of some future archeologist digging through our landfills, finding a narrow band of dense plastic bottles that can be dated to the twenty-first century, and concluding that this was an early form of intentional carbon sequestration practiced when we learned that our carbon dioxide emissions were going to radically change the climate.

In any case, it is getting harder and more expensive to simply dump our garbage in landfills. The number of landfills in the United States has dropped since the late 1980s from nearly 8,000 to under 2,000 as landfills have filled up and closed in recent years. And as the costs of disposing of our garbage have risen, new efforts have been launched to try to reduce the volume of waste and, especially, to recycle and reclaim reusable materials such as aluminum, paper, organic matter, and a few kinds of plastic, including PET.

As criticism of bottled water has grown, we hear over and over from the bottled water industry that plastic PET bottles are fully recyclable. "The bottles our member companies produce are 100% recyclable," blared a full-page ad taken out by the International Bottled Water Association in the *New York Times* and the *San Francisco Chronicle* in August 2007. "Our water bottles—as well as all of our product containers like aluminum cans and glass bottles—are 100 percent recyclable," said Craig Stevens, spokesman for the American Beverage Association.[6] "Our Eco-Shape bottle is 100% recyclable," touts Nestlé on their Ozarka, Poland Springs, Deer Park, and Arrowhead websites.

Ah. Not to quibble, but "recyclable" is not the same as "recycled." Water bottles are almost all recyclable, and yet most of them are never recycled. In 2007 the National Association for PET Container Resources (or NAPCOR) reported that over 5.6 billion pounds of PET bottles and jars were available for recycling, but only 1.4 billion pounds of PET were actually recycled—an overall recycling rate of under 25 percent. This is higher than recent years, but well below the rates of plastic recycling in the mid-1990s, when as many as 40 percent of PET bottles were recycled.7 According to the nonprofit Container Recycling Institute, recycling rates for PET *water* bottles are even lower than for other PET containers. The United States actually recycles far fewer plastic water bottles, and less plastic overall, than just about anything else in the waste stream we generate.

So what if I want to recycle my PET water bottle? Like a growing number of households, I have a number of options: I can return it to a nearby recycling center at a grocery store; I can take it to Berkeley's central recycling plant; or my son can do his chores and put it out on our curb in a separate blue bin late on Wednesday night with our other recycling materials. Thursday morning, that plastic bottle, along with the rest of my recycling, is picked up by a truck operated by Berkeley's nonprofit recycling program—the Ecology Center. The Ecology Center has a contract with the city to collect and recycle all paper, cardboard, aluminum, glass, and two kinds of plastic bottles, PET and HDPE (the ones with the number 1 and number 2 plastics logos on them). All the paper goes into one container on the Ecology Center trucks and all the other materials go into another, to be sorted at the recycling center. Some recycling programs will accept all plastics, which greatly increases the volume of plastic that is collected but reduces the value, since the recycler can often get more money for clean streams of PET or HDPE than for streams of mixed plastics. In particular, recyclers have nicknamed polyvinyl chloride (number 3) "Satan's Resin" because of its toxic properties and completely unrecyclable nature, and they try hard to avoid having it contaminate recyclable materials.

In early 2009 I went down to the Ecology Center facility in Berkeley to see where my plastic goes. The day I visited the Center, they were paying individuals a healthy 96 cents a pound for PET bottles and 54 cents a pound for HDPE bottles, which helps explains why all the high-quality plastics are often scavenged from my curb-side recycled bins in the middle of the night before the Center's trucks can collect them. All together the Center collects around 8,000 tons of recycling a year from over 35,000 households and thousands of businesses, around one-fifth of which consists of drink containers.

The recycling system in place in Berkeley is relatively simple, using real people and straightforward technology to sort the recycling into a few basic categories. "Separation is key," Andrew Schneider, Berkeley's recycling specialist, told me. "Berkeley has a reputation for producing clean streams," which are vital for getting good contracts with material resellers who don't want to buy mixed or contaminated materials. In Berkeley, a magnet pulls out tin-plated steel cans and other iron-based materials. Aluminum cans are grabbed by hand and tossed down another chute. Plastics are separated into three streams: PET, HDPE, and other plastics. Glass is sorted by color into brown, green, and clear streams.

The separated PET is crushed, perforated, baled into cubes roughly a meter on a side, and loaded into a shipping container. Berkeley has a contract with a few plastic exporters or domestic reprocessors, and every day or so a container full of PET bales gets placed on a truck and shipped to a plastic exporter, who in turn sends it to be recycled where it is either cleaned, chopped, or shredded into little "flakes" and turned back into new feedstock for PET, or crushed, shredded, and made into a wide range of polyester products, including carpet, clothing, automotive parts, strapping material, and plastic toys. In all, Berkeley sends around six tons of PET a week to plastics recyclers—much of it used water bottles.

Berkeley's recycling system is called "single stream," since residents don't have to separate out glass, plastic, and aluminum into different containers. Some cities require that the homeowner or business carefully sort materials before they are picked up, but this requires trucks with five, or six, or even seven separate containers, and even then, the central facility has to have a way to deal with blended materials from lazy recyclers. In some cities, the separation of recyclable materials from garbage is increasingly being done by machines in a "materials recovery facility" or MRF ("merf"). The technology for MRFs is rapidly improving and sophisticated systems can do more sophisticated sorting. New machines that automatically sort PET from other plastics dramatically increase plastic recovery rates while reducing labor costs. Smart MRFs, for example, can even differentiate among different colors of PET, HDPE milk jugs and water containers, mixed colored HDPE containers, such as detergent containers, or shampoo bottles, and they can separate out plastics numbers 3 through 7 to be sold separately or as a mix.

There are dozens of businesses that buy recycled plastic and repackage it for sale to domestic recyclers or for export. Of all PET collected for recycling in the United States, half went to the fourteen reclamation plants operated in the U.S. by domestic recyclers. The other half is exported. Demand is especially intense in China. In an example of the bizarre economics that define the modern world, most of our recycled bottles end up in giant bundles stuffed onto container ships heading for Asia. The Chinese find it cheaper to buy our plastic garbage, ship it across the entire Pacific Ocean, and use it to make stuff to ship back here, than to make virgin PET from petroleum. And they can't get enough of our plastic garbage. At times, Chinese recyclers have found themselves in bidding wars in the ports of Long Beach and Oakland, California, competing for bundles of plastic garbage coming from all over the country.

The economics of recycling are complicated and variable, affected by oil and energy prices, demand for materials, and even the overall state of the economy, as well as whether a state has a bottle bill that supports recycling programs. A high price for oil raises transportation costs and makes it more expensive to ship recycled materials overseas, yet it also raises the cost of virgin PET, making recycled materials more attractive. Some countries require that PET bottles contain at least some recycled materials in order to encourage markets for recycled plastic, while other countries ban the use of recycled materials for food containers because of fear of contamination. At times recyclers, who are often required by law to collect plastics, have actually had to pay exporters to take mixed bags of plastic when the market for recycling weakened, as happened in the economic collapse in late 2008. The once red-hot global demand for recycled plastic plunged and containers of plastic scrap began piling up at Chinese ports as importers failed to claim the goods. Demand for plastic resin also plummeted as demand for toys and clothes made from PET dried up.

Right now, we can't recycle all of our PET water bottles. Traditional recycling programs were not designed with plastics in mind, but were focused instead on getting consumers to bring back empty containers made from aluminum and glass. The very first bottle bill was passed in Oregon in 1971 with the simple idea that you pay a nickel deposit on a glass or aluminum container when you buy it and you get your nickel back when you return it. The idea of putting a price on garbage was radical, and yet it was an undisputed success. The year after it was implemented, recycling rates for glass and aluminum in Oregon went from 25 percent to more than 90 percent. In states with bottle bills, recycling rates range from 65 to 95 percent, substantially higher than in the states without deposit laws. Yet despite this record, the powerful beverage industry and grocery lobbies have successfully fought the expansion of bottle bill laws. Only eleven of the fifty states have bottle bills: California, Connecticut, Delaware, Hawaii, Maine, Massachusetts, Michigan, New York, Iowa, Oregon, and Vermont.

Moreover, none of the existing bottle bills include adjustments for inflation, and a nickel in 1971 is worth about a penny today. As a result, recycling rates are falling, even in states with bottle bills. And how many of us actually get our nickel back? We typically pay the deposit when we buy the container, but if we throw it away or put it out at the curb for recycling, the beverage industry often gets to keep the money—hundreds of millions of dollars a year. Even worse, almost no bottle bills include deposits for bottled water, which barely existed when the first bills were passed in 1971, and recent efforts to close this loophole and expand the definitions in existing laws to include bottled water have been regularly defeated. In 2009, years of effort by New York State to make its bottle bill apply to water bottles finally succeeded, making it only the sixth state to include a deposit on water bottles. As a result, U. S. water bottle recycling rates are far below those of other beverage cans and bottles.

Some countries do much better. Comprehensive container deposit regulations are in place in countries like Australia, Canada, Denmark, Germany, Norway, and Sweden. In some of these countries, plastic bottle recycling rates can approach 90 percent. In Switzerland, there are bottle bins at every supermarket with separate slots for clear, green, and brown glass and for plastic bottles. As a result, 80 percent of plastic PET bottles are recycled there, far higher than the overall European average of 40 percent.[8] Some countries are implementing "take-back" programs that require companies to either reduce waste volumes or accept packaging waste from their products for recycling or disposal. In June 2003 the Pollution Control Board of West Bengal, India, told bottle producers that they were now responsible for collecting and recycling used bottles.[9]

Another way to boost recycling rates is to require that plastic bottles contain more recycled content. Existing markets are capable of using far more recycled PET if regulators require it or manufacturers voluntary commit to using recycled PET. Small actions can have big effects. In 2004 the use of recycled PET in non-food containers tripled in the United States, solely as a result of California enforcing a law (the "Rigid Plastics Packaging Container Law") that requires the use of 25 percent post-consumer resin content in non-food packaging products.[10]

The major water bottlers could, in theory, use recycled PET to make all their bottles. They've made noises about this over the years: In 1990 both Coca-Cola and PepsiCo made voluntary commitments to use up to 25 percent recycled PET in their beverage bottles, but quickly abandoned those commitments. In 2000 Coca-Cola announced their intention to reach a target of 10 percent recycled PET use in beverage containers and PepsiCo followed suit in 2002. Both companies claim to have temporarily reached that target by 2005, before again backing off their efforts. In 2008 Coca-Cola again announced their intention, this time by 2010, to boost the recycled PET content of their bottles to 10 percent. To help meet their goals, in 2009 Coca-Cola opened the world's largest plastic "bottle-to-bottle" recycling plant in Spartanburg, South Carolina. This plant will eventually be capable of producing around 100 million pounds of recycled PET plastic for use in new bottles each year,[11] though the company continues to oppose new state container deposit bills (or "Forced Deposit Bills," as the company characterizes them).[12] In Great Britain in 2007, two beverage makers, Innocent Drinks and Ribena, both announced their intention to use 100 percent recycled PET for their drink containers.[13] Until these efforts lead to higher recycling rates, the number of PET water bottles that end up in our landfills is likely to remain high.

If it is hard to boost recycling rates, perhaps the amount of plastic used to produce each bottle can be reduced. This is the main approach taken by the bottled water industry in its efforts to counter criticism of the high environmental and energy costs of producing PET. The concept is called "lightweighting" by the packaging industry (in a particularly striking example of verbifying a noun or adjective). Lightweighting reduces the cost of production, the energy required for shipping, and the mass of plastic in landfills. Beverage manufacturers have achieved some remarkable success with this in other areas: the food industry has reduced the weight of aluminum cans by 26 percent between 1975 and 2005. Steel cans now weigh 40 percent of what they did in 1970. Glass containers are half the weight they were in 1990.[14]

The same trend is underway in the plastics industry. The weight of PET bottles has fallen by 25 percent since 1977, and new efforts are underway to make them even lighter. In the course of work I've done evaluating the energy implications of plastics production, I surveyed the weight of PET water bottles. The average weight of 45 different bottles was 44 grams per liter of volume. But nearly a dozen newer bottles now weigh less than 25 grams per liter. Nestlé's is particularly proud of their efforts in this area. In 2007 they introduced the "Eco-shape®" half-liter bottle weighing 12.5 grams, and the French packaging company Sidel has developed a half-liter "NoBottle™" that weighs in at 9.9 grams. While the trend toward lightweighting will continue, there are structural limits to how light and thin a PET water bottle can be made. In the end lightweighting does nothing to increase recycling rates or reduce the actual volume and numbers of bottles ending up in landfills.

In addition to recycling and lightweighting, the volume of plastics going to landfills can be reduced through incineration. More countries and municipalities are burning solid wastes that cannot be, or haven't been, recycled or composted. Incinerators can reduce municipal solid waste volumes substantially—by as much as 70 to 90 percent according to some estimates—while simultaneously generating electricity and heat. Modern incinerators can produce energy with very low emissions of pollutants, unlike early waste incinerators that spewed all sorts of nasty things into the air over nearby populations. In 2007 the United States had 87 waste-to-energy plants capable of producing 2,700 megawatts of power and handling about 13 percent of our trash. The Japanese have also moved strongly in this area, actually reducing efforts to recycle plastics because they find that they get far more energy burning the plastic than would be saved by recycling it. A trade-off of this approach, however, is that burning plastic creates carbon dioxide—the principal gas responsible for global warming—and other air pollutants, converting a solid waste problem into an air pollution problem.

Then why not create "green," environmentally friendly bottles made of a biodegradable material as a way of reducing the problem of billions of plastic bottles that will last forever in our landfills? Part of the challenge is producing a food-grade container with all of the strengths and advantages of PET without the liabilities. A few possible materials have been tried, and entrepreneurial bottlers are beginning to sell bottled water in them, though with little success. One such alternative to PET is polylactic acid (PLA), or polylactide. PLA can be made from almost any starchy vegetable, including potatoes, beets, and corn. The largest producer of PLA is NatureWorks, a joint venture between giant corn producer Cargill and Teijin Ltd. of China. Cargill's NatureWorks unit then sells PLA to a variety of food packagers, including Walmart, Wild Oats Markets, Del Monte, and Newman's Own.

Unfortunately, PLA has some serious liabilities of its own. First of all, the stuff is not really very biodegradable. Cargill claims that PLA will degrade rapidly in certain environments into carbon dioxide, water, and organic material. Those conditions, however, are high heat, high moisture, and the presence of certain micro-organisms— conditions not commonly found in landfills. NatureWorks has acknowledged that PLA dumped in a landfill will probably last as long as a PET bottle.[15] No advantage there.

Even worse, recyclers are afraid that the presence of PLA bottles in PET recycling streams will contaminate them. Separating PLA from PET is hard to do. While pure PET has a relatively high value, recyclers consider it contaminated—and the market value drops considerably—if more than around 1 percent of the bottles are not PET. This can worsen the already marginal economics of recycling centers, where PET often makes up an important part of the revenue stream. Other questions about PLA arise. How should it be labeled? Should PLA be made from corn or is corn too valuable as a food product—a worry made even more serious by the recent push for corn-based ethanol and growing global food shortages.

Because of these problems, a coalition of recycling organizations and local recyclers asked NatureWorks in October 2006 for a moratorium on any expansion of using PLA for bottles until the bio-resin's recyclability has been demonstrated. The members of the coalition include a mix of recycling and community waste-management groups, such as the Plastic Redesign Project, Eco-Cycle, Eureka Recycling, the Ecology Center in California, the Institute for Local Self-Reliance, the Center for a Competitive Waste Industry, and the GrassRoots Recycling Network. Eric Lombardi, president of the Grassroots Recycling Network, said that if NatureWorks doesn't cooperate, "We will educate the public to avoid products bottled in PLA."[16]

Despite the opposition to PLA, NatureWorks is continuing its aggressive expansion efforts. A growing number of water bottlers have adopted PLA for packaging water. In 2006 a company called Biota offered what they claimed was "the World's First bottled water/beverage packaged in a Planet Friendly bottle," and they continue to sell water in PLA bottles. In 2008 Primo Water Corporation of Winston-Salem, North Carolina, started offering water in 16.9-ounce bottles made from NatureWork's PLA.[17] The industry has also launched a conference to push the use of PLA in bottles. The first one, held in Hamburg, Germany, in September 2007, drew 100 industry participants from 25 countries and led to a major "world congress" on PLA in the fall of 2008 in Munich.[18]

There are other alternatives to PET under development. In May 2009 Coca-Cola announced that they were going to test a new "PlantBottle™" that is a mix of plastic, sugar cane, and molasses, calling it more "environmentally friendly." Beginning in late 2009 they will test the bottle with Dasani bottled water and some of their carbonated brands. This material appears to be PET, but with some of the petroleum-based components of PET replaced with more natural biomass materials. This composition can still be recycled using traditional PET recycling methods without contaminating the waste stream, but it may not degrade any faster in our landfills.

In the meantime, while we invest enormous sums of money in new materials for bottled water, our investment in convenient public water is going to waste. Most public fountains in London and Paris and our other cities and towns are gone or disconnected. New public buildings, like the University of Central Florida's new stadium, are increasingly built without them. And existing fountains are not adequately cleaned or maintained. A survey of university campuses in Canada reveals the extent of this trend. A third of survey respondents noticed a drop in the number of water fountains on campus, while nearly half said they noticed delays in repairing broken fountains. One respondent from Brock University in Ontario, Canada, said, "In new buildings on campus, there are no water fountains, only Pepsi machines, and the water fountains that do exist are sparse and in inaccessible places." At Carleton University in Ottawa, the Physical Plant department issued a directive saying that fountains that could not easily be repaired would not be replaced.[19] In June 2008, the associate vice president of land and building services at the University of British Columbia was quoted as saying that because drinking water fountains are not required under B.C. building codes there is no obligation to install them.[20] A similar national poll of a thousand Australians found the same problem. Nine out of ten people said they didn't know where to find a local water fountain (which Australians call "bubblers"). Eighty-five percent said they worried about the cleanliness and safety of drinking from fountains. And 80 percent said there weren't enough fountains in their city. "As far as the public are concerned, public water bubblers have disappeared off the map," said Jon Dee, an organizer of the Bottled Water Alliance, which commissioned the poll. "The lack of uniform signage for bubblers and the concerns that people have about the upkeep and quality of public bubblers are significant—they're two of the reasons why Australians are spending half a billion dollars on bottled water every year."[21]

In August 2005 Andrew Ferguson wrote a scathing report on the state of the Washington, D.C., mall. Among other things, he noted the complete lack of water: "If you want a vision of hell, look here: the national mall in Washington, D.C., at noon on a summer's day . . . hey, where are the water fountains?"[22] In New York's Central Park, even today, there are still 150 drinking fountains, but many no longer function, or they are dirty and ignored. The Park's public watchdog group regularly gives the fountains a failing grade, describing them as "plagued by maintenance, safety, and structural challenges. Even when drinking fountains provide water with sufficient pressure, users frequently find trash, mold, and severe leaks."[23] In schools around the country, water fountains are scorned or turned off because of fears of contamination. Instead, children arrive at school with expensive single-serve plastic "Aquapods" tucked in their lunches and backpacks—little throwaway water bottles marketed by Nestlé to parents as a convenient and healthy alternative to the soda and juice containers that have also replaced milk cartons in our children's school lunches. Or students buy bottled water from the vending machines aggressively promoted to school districts by beverage companies.

We've become more reluctant to drink from public water fountains, and the convenient availability of bottled water has further reduced public demands for fountains. Who hasn't seen trucks driving around our streets delivering bottled water to homes or schools or businesses, or hand carts stacked high with bottled water being delivered to outlets in our airports, malls, or convenience stores? If any movement away from bottled water is going to succeed, there must be good, safe, and conveniently available alternatives.

The irony is that the more bottled water we buy, the more invested in it we become and the more susceptible we become to industry efforts to convince consumers that bottled water is not a luxury, but a necessity. Part of that effort is their campaign to vilify tap water, but another part is their use of the classic tools of advertising and marketing to make bottled water attractive—tools that have proven so successful in our commercial, product-driven society. If you're peddling something that looks, tastes, and smells the same as your competitors, you have to find other ways to make your product stand out and to convince consumers to spend their money on what you're selling.

CHAPTER 8

Selling Bottled Water: The Modern Medicine Show

Advertising is the art of convincing people to spend money they don't have for something they don't need.
— Will Rogers

It may be necessary to fool people for their own good. . . . Average intelligence is surprisingly low. It is so much more effectively guided by its subconscious impulses and instincts than by its reason.
— John Benson, President of the American Association of Advertising Agencies[1]

I CONSIDER MYSELF a pretty savvy consumer. My wife and I tried to teach our children from a young age how to question advertisements and to understand how ads manipulate our emotions and play on our dreams. But despite my inherent skepticism, I can't begin to count the number of thirty-second advertisements, for things I don't own and would never buy, that still manage to bring tears to my eyes. A good advertiser can sell us something we don't want or need. A truly great advertiser can convince us to pay a thousand times more than we're already paying for something we already have. Like water.

The art of advertising is really the art of manipulating images and beliefs with the tools of illusion, desire, ambiguity, and innuendo for the purpose of selling something. This isn't necessarily either good or bad: People with limited time to shop and short attention spans are often faced with a vast array of competing and indistinguishable products. And when the product is bottled water, all the special tricks of advertisers are needed. Indeed, bottled water advertisers don't try to sell water: They sell youth, health, beauty, romance, status, image, and, of course, the old standbys, sex and fear. Typical slogans from some bottled water campaigns tell the tale:

Can't live without it. (Dasani)
Far from pollution. Far from acid rain. Far from industrial waste. (Fiji Artesian Water)
Sip smarter. Live Longer. (Poland Spring)
Your natural source of youth. (Evian)
My slimness partner. (Contrex)
Trust in every drop. (Kinley)
Cleansed inside, beautiful outside. (Rocchetta)
The oldest way to stay young. (Infinity Water)
Pleasure within you. (Agua Castello)

The history of marketing water with extravagant and questionable claims goes back centuries. As early as 1630 a Massachusetts merchant was fined for claiming his special water would cure scurvy.[2] When disease was widespread, medicine rudimentary, and doctors rare, quackery and medical mysticism abounded as people desperately searched for cures to their ailments.

By the late 1800s newspapers, magazines, and mail-order catalogues in Europe and the United States were packed with advertisements for remedies that were often therapeutically useless and sometimes outright dangerous, containing alcohol, opium, cocaine, and even—literally—snake oil. Ironically, some snake oils actually have therapeutic effects, but over time the moniker "snake oil" has come to describes products with both exaggerated marketing and questionable benefits.[3] In rural regions of the United States, traveling medicine shows first captured people's attention with entertaining magic, juggling and circus acts, comedians, music, and storytelling, and then captured their money with salesmen and con artists pitching magic waters, patent medicines, mysterious nostrums, and miracle cures. "Cure All Diseases" claimed the bottles of water, sulfuric acid, and red wine peddled by the famous fraud, William Radam. "Restore life in the event of sudden death," claimed "Dr." Sibley's "Reanimating Solar Tincture." An English quack, "Dr. Solomon," offered Cordial Balm of Gilead as a cure for almost everything, especially venereal diseases. His concoction turned out to be water with brandy and herbs.

Due to growing complaints of fraud and false advertising, Congress felt pressure in the early 1870s to authorize the postmaster general to fight con artists who were using the mail to both advertise and deliver ineffective health remedies. Initially, efforts focused on stopping any "scheme or device for obtaining money through the mails by means of false or fraudulent pretenses, representations, or promises."4 By the turn of the century, frauds involving "quack medicines" were so prevalent that the public began to call on the government to strengthen laws to protect the public, and on June 30, 1906, President Theodore Roosevelt signed the Pure Food and Drugs Act—the first national law to offer rules and regulations to counter the proliferation of ineffective, contaminated, or dangerous foods and drugs.5 The law required manufacturers to use honest labels about contents and restricted advertisers from making unsubstantiated health or medical claims. In particular, labels could not contain any "statement, design, or device" that was "false or misleading in any particular."6 In July 1906 the *New York Times* editorialized that the law was a vital effort to protect "the purity and honesty of the food and medicines of the people."7

In his wonderful 1967 history of medical quackery, *The Medical Messiahs*, James Harvey Young described how conflicting court opinions and loopholes in the 1906 law itself permitted false and misleading labels to continue to flourish. In August 1912 Congress went back and strengthened the law with an amendment that declared a food or drug to be misbranded "if its package or label shall bear or contain any statement, design, or device regarding the curative or therapeutic effect of such an article or any of the ingredients or substances contained therein, which is false and fraudulent."[8]

Under President Woodrow Wilson, the Federal Trade Commission statute of 1914 added more protections against fraud and false advertising. By this point, even some advertisers wanted government help to curtail fraudulent claims because of the fear that the public would begin to distrust all advertisements. The Associated Advertising Clubs of America wrote that the "value of advertisements depends largely upon the credence placed in them by the public" and they lobbied in favor of state laws banning especially "pernicious practices."[9] Despite these efforts, wild claims continued to appear in print and radio advertising. By the outbreak of the First World War, even groups like the Proprietary Association, which normally lobbied against restrictions on the food and drug industry, noted: "Advertisements that a short time ago were rejected with disdain are now accepted with alacrity if not cheerfulness."[10]

Advertising expanded enormously after the First World War as new industries were created, personal consumption grew, women became major buyers of goods and services, and businesses eagerly sought out new markets. Advertisers knew they didn't have to sell a product directly—they could sell emotion. In 1927 Mr. John Benson, soon to be president of the American Association of Advertising Agencies, wrote: "It may be necessary to fool people for their own good. . . . Average intelligence is surprisingly low. It is so much more effectively guided by its subconscious impulses and instincts than by its reason."[11]

Pro-business governments in place after the First World War continued to rely on self-regulation, voluntary efforts, and cooperative agreements with businesses. During the 1920s the National Vigilance Committee, which ultimately became the National Better Business Bureau (NBBB), worked to promote industry-wide, albeit voluntary, cooperation over advertising practices. The NBBB produced public warnings and bulletins covering a wide range of products, such as diet remedies, radioactive waters, and so-called health foods.

This voluntary approach simply didn't work. By the mid-1920s even some in the business community began to acknowledge that legal and regulatory remedies and a reliance on voluntary self-control on the part of manufacturers and advertisers were inadequate to the scope of the problem. William E. Humphrey, a pro-business appointee to the Federal Trade Commission, railed against the "lunatic fringe" in the advertising sector.[12] Americans, Humphrey said in a blistering 1926 speech to the National Petroleum Association, "are annually robbed of hundreds of millions of dollars through these fake advertisements. All of these prey upon the weak and the unfortunate, the ignorant and the credulous. There is no viler class of criminal known among men."[13]

The financial crises of the Great Depression made things worse. Shrinking markets and tighter budgets drove even honest manufacturers to use advertising methods and claims they had previously shunned in order to try to sell their goods. Newspapers and magazines were increasingly unable or unwilling to evaluate advertising claims for fear of losing revenue. "So far as advertising goes, we are fallen on evil days," said H. A. Batten, an East Coast advertising executive in the July 1932 issue of *The Atlantic Monthly*.[14]

Every time the government tried to crack down on fraud and misrepresentation, industry and its allies quickly pushed through new loopholes, mounted legal challenges, or eviscerated enforcement powers. And even when an occasional ruling or enforcement action succeeded, the offending parties often simply slithered away, reopened under a different name (or even the same name), and kept right on doing business. And the prohibition against outright lies has never been much of a barrier to advertisers when enforcement is inconsistent and weak.

The evil days of snake oil salesmen and medicine shows are still with us, and bottled water is often the product being hawked. A vast array of bottled waters are being peddled as miracle cures for all kinds of ailments and modern worries. Fraudulent claims made about the magical benefits of some bottled waters are the same kind of claims made for the magical benefits of patent medicines in the early part of the twentieth century. What do I choose? The bottled water that promises to make me slim? Or the bottled water that promises to complement my desire for a healthy lifestyle? How about the one that offers the hint of sex? Oh yeah! Or the one that offers freedom from fear of disease, contamination, and illness that will result if I drink my tap water? Or perhaps the bottled water whose molecules have been mysteriously rearranged to offer health and emotional salvation? The gullible consumer can find all of these things, with no sign of the regulators who should be protecting us.

A New Alchemy

If you can come up with two or more pseudoscientific, hyphenated words—some of them adjectives and one of them "water"—you too can market bottled water as a miracle cure. Ionized water. Vibrationally charged interactive water. Alkalized water. Energy-enhanced water infused with luck or love. Clustered water. Weight-loss "skinny" water. Super-oxygenated water. Magnetized water. Rhythm-structured water. Scalarwave-imprinted, hexagonally-structured water. Positive-energy water. Improved fractal-design water. Water infused with Reiki energy. These are just some of the magical bottled waters pushed on ignorant consumers or people with real health concerns who don't know where else to turn for help. Pseudoscientific claims for bottled waters can be found in brochures, health stores, and magazines, and especially on the Internet. As use of the Internet has exploded, we are seeing a proliferation of websites that make explicit, unsubstantiated, outlandish, and often blatantly fraudulent claims about the health benefits of bottled waters. And we're sucking it up by the gallon.

Some of these claims are beginning to draw the attention and ire of consumer advocates and debunkers of pseudoscience. Skeptic P. Z. Myers in his blog "Pharyngula" describes claims about "clustered waters" as "pure unadulterated bullshit" peddled by "greased weasels."[15] Famous stage magician and debunker of pseudoscientific nonsense James Randi calls unproven bottled water claims "deception" and "thievery," and he has challenged some bottlers to prove their more outlandish assertions and win a million-dollar prize he has offered to anyone capable of proving a paranormal or pseudoscientific claim under laboratory conditions. So far his million dollars is safe.

But where are the federal regulators whose job it is to protect consumers from these kinds of false claims? Didn't we win this fight more than a hundred years ago, when America put in place laws to guard our foods and drugs against fraud and to end false, unregulated advertising? Nowhere to be seen. Institutions created a century ago to protect the public, like the Food and Drug Administration and FTC, were never strong to begin with, and one of the legacies of the anti-government, anti-regulation, anti-enforcement movement of the past few decades has been to further weaken consumer protections to the point that misleading, unproven claims are rarely challenged.

The Internet has made it much easier both to make such claims and to spread them widely. In theory, advertising on the Internet is subject to the same laws as advertising in newspapers, magazines, radio, and television. In reality, advertising on the Internet is less well monitored and consumer protection laws are less frequently enforced. As a result, consumers are far more vulnerable to misleading information and outright fraud than we would have been just a decade ago, when the channels of information reaching us were more limited and more regulated. When advertisers worked solely through traditional media, monitoring was easier, oversight and enforcement more manageable. Today, new mechanisms for fraud develop far faster and are more nimble than government regulation and oversight. More of us get more of our information, advertising, and products online than ever before, from websites that may be put up for a few dollars and managed from outside of our traditional regulatory and political borders, far from the reach of our legal systems.

Who Is Supposed to Be Protecting the Bottled Water Consumer?

The bottled water industry seems to produce more than its share of cons. The regulation of even legitimate bottled water advertising and marketing in the United States has always been hazy and inconsistent, with overlapping or conflicting jurisdictions. General advertising fraud is monitored and regulated by the Federal Trade Commission (FTC). The Food and Drug Administration (FDA) regulates food and health products, including bottled water. General Internet crime falls partly under the control of the Criminal Division of the Department of Justice, especially the Computer Crime and Intellectual Property Section (CCIPS).

But the Internet Fraud Complaint Center (IFCC) is a partnership of the Federal Bureau of Investigation (FBI) and the National White Collar Crime Center. Separately, the FBI, the Drug Enforcement Agency, and the Department of Justice have recently focused on online ventures that sell or promote health-care products. Some states run their own programs for addressing advertising or business fraud through state agencies or the Better Business Bureau, which maintains the National Advertising Review Council, a voluntary industry oversight group. Nongovernment organizations also play a role in the United States, such as the National Consumer League, which manages the website Internet Fraud Watch.*

Two basic principles of FTC regulation apply to advertising wherever it appears. An ad or claim must be truthful and not misleading; and before disseminating an ad, advertisers must have adequate substantiation to support objective product claims. The FTC defines substantiation as "competent and reliable scientific" evidence consisting of "tests, studies, or other scientific evidence that has been conducted and evaluated according to standards that experts in the field accept as accurate and reliable. Under the FTC Act, anecdotal reports, articles in popular magazines, opinions, and inadequately controlled open label studies are not considered adequate substantiation and cannot be used as substitutes for scientific support."** But these federal agencies are failing in their basic missions. Not only are they failing to protect us from contamination, as we've seen, they are not even protecting us from obvious charlatans peddling false claims and pseudoscience about bottled water.

---

* See http://www.fraud.org/internet/intstat.htm.

** See http://www.ftc.gov/bcp/reports/weightloss.pdf, p. 25; see also http://www.ftc.gov/os/2005/04/050411weightlosssurvey04.pdf.

Even if a scam is successfully challenged in one jurisdiction, it will often pop up somewhere else a short time later.

For example, what does all our regulatory brainpower and legal policing authority do when confronted with a website that makes the following claims?

> After many years of research and conscious deliberation, Dr. Emoto is able to provide the world with a stable, consumable hexagonal water, imprinted with frequencies to support creativity, balance, and conscious awareness. . . . There is no question that hexagonally structured water provides more rapid hydration. . . . Dr. Emoto's Hexagonal Water is more easily assimilated at the cellular level. It may be one of the best ways to overcome dehydration and protect your body from the symptoms of disease and premature aging. Within minutes, Dr. Emoto's water moves into the cells, taking nutrients and expelling metabolic wastes more efficiently than bottled water."[16]

So what do our regulators do about this? The answer is, nothing. Most bottled water scams should be easy targets for FTC or FDA action. But understaffed federal agencies and an atmosphere of regulatory minimalism leave most of them untouched.

In 2007 I started to track down legal actions taken against fraudulent bottled water claims by the FTC and the FDA. After hours of fruitless Internet searching, phone calls to regulatory agencies, and data requests to the FTC, I filed a Freedom of Information Act request in late 2007. After ten months of back-and-forth, the FTC finally sent me their response: There have been fewer than half a dozen actions against bottled water and almost none against misleading health claims.

All of this would be less of a concern if these kinds of claims were rare. They aren't. While most of the big corporate bottlers are careful to avoid making misleading assertions, unsubstantiated and even outright false claims are promulgated by literally dozens, if not hundreds, of water bottlers around the world. And these would often be amusing rather than dangerous, except that they take money from people to line the pockets of liars and cheats, and they may prevent people from seeking out legitimate medical treatments for real ailments in the hopes of finding miracle cures from a plastic bottle of magic water.

Here are a few of the classic pseudoscientific distortions regularly offered to the public by bottled water hucksters.

Oxygen Water

Oxygen is good. We breathe it. So what could be better than drinking water specially infused with extra oxygen? The idea that adding oxygen to water offers health benefits has led to a broad set of scams offering oxygenated or "superoxygenated" bottled water at dozens of websites. Other companies offer special oxygen "coolers" that one can buy to add oxygen to your own water. For example, you can buy a special "Millennium Oxygen Cooler" for just $995 or an "Oxygenated Bottled Water Cooler Table Top with cold oxygen water dispenser" for $695 (plus shipping).

Such companies claim a variety of health and performance benefits for their water. Some sellers allege that special oxygenated waters can enhance brain function, increase muscle performance, promote healthier, younger looking skin, accelerate the absorption of vitamins and nutrients, and fight bacteria and viruses. "Perk up the natural way with a glass of oxygenated water from the O_2 cooler! Adding oxygen to your bloodstream has been proven to speed up metabolism, strengthen your immune system, increase energy, create younger-looking skin, and even enhance brain function for clearer, more alert thinking," one website claimed in early 2009, implying of course that their product provided exactly these benefits.[17] Another website argues that we should oxygenate our water because "We are simply NOT getting as much oxygen as our human bodies were designed for! . . . Scientists were stunned to discover that atmospheric oxygen content in ancient times measured twice as high as that of today: It was 38 percent 10,000 years ago, compared to the 21 percent of today, getting lower and lower due to pollution and industrialization."[18]

Scientists would indeed be stunned to discover this, since while the composition of the atmosphere has varied dramatically over the eons, atmospheric chemists believe that the level of oxygen in the atmosphere has remained steady for millions of years and is close to what it has been since the emergence of modern *homo sapiens* a hundred thousand years ago. More important, the very small natural variations from place to place make no difference to our health.[19]

Another website writes: "We are able to increase the oxygen content of our Premium Bottled Water by 700%—the maximum amount of oxygen possible! That's seven times more oxygen!"[20] Actually, a 700 percent increase would be eight times more oxygen, not seven, but my real quibble here is with the company's scientific and physiological illiteracy, not their innumeracy. First, while it is possible to put extra oxygen into bottled water, it doesn't stay there long once you open the bottle. Second, even if you were to quickly drink water with extra oxygen there is no proven health benefit, nor alteration in the taste. In properly designed and independent scientific tests, no health or performance difference between plain tap water and water with extra oxygen has ever been shown. On the contrary, studies consistently show no benefit of oxygenated water.[21] In a detailed scientific study published in the *Journal of the American Medical Association* (*JAMA*) in 2003, the scientists noted while bottlers sometimes claim that their bottled water has 600 or 700 percent more oxygen than tap water, extra oxygen doesn't stay in solution for long. Of the five brands of oxygenated water tested in the *JAMA* study, one had no more oxygen than regular tap water, and the other four had only slightly elevated levels—the highest had 80 ml of O_2 in a twelve-ounce bottle. A single normal human breath contains 100 ml of O_2. The scientists note:

Thus, a single breath of air contains more O_2 than a bottle of oxygenated water. Given that hemoglobin is already nearly saturated with O_2 during air breathing, and that only a small amount of additional O_2 can be dissolved in plasma, it is not surprising that oxygenated water did not improve maximal exercise performance.

No physical or taste benefits were found either. "There were no significant differences in exercise results after participants drank either oxygenated or tap water for any measured variables. Furthermore, the participants were unable to identify oxygenated water by taste."[22]

The final scientific *coup de grâce* to the idea of oxygenated water is that even if you manage to drink water with a bit more oxygen in it, it goes to the stomach, not the lungs. Yet it is the lungs that transmit oxygen to the bloodstream. If you really want more oxygen in your blood, take a deep breath. Or, as Howard Knuttgen, PhD and editor-in-chief of the *Georgia Tech Sports Medicine & Performance Newsletter*, said in 2001 in a review of the benefits of oxygenated water, all that may result from drinking this stuff is "an expensive burp" and, I might note, a thinner wallet, since you can pay $35 a case or more for this stuff.[23] Despite this basic science, you can still buy dozens of versions of oxygenated water today sold by companies that continue to make a wide range of health claims. They even maintain that drinking oxygenated water can promote "clearer thinking," which could be a good thing for the people who buy it, if only it actually worked.

The closest the FTC or FDA has ever come to challenging these enhanced oxygen claims was an FTC case filed in March 1999 against Rose Creek Health Products Inc. and Staff of Life Inc., marketers of something called Vitamin O (O for oxygen). The company claimed in print and online that Vitamin O drops (drops of their magic liquid that you buy to put in your own water) were a way to enhance the oxygen content of water and that they offered, among

other things, health benefits, including the potential to cure or prevent cancer, heart disease, and lung disease. The FTC found that
Vitamin O was nothing more than drops of salt water,[24] and contrary to claims, does not allow oxygen molecules to be absorbed
through the gastrointestinal system, does not prevent or treat any
physical ailment or disease, does not have a beneficial effect on
human health, has not been proven effective by medical or scientific
research, and was not developed, as claimed, by NASA for use of
astronauts.[25] The FTC received a $375,000 judgment issued against
the manufacturers in 2000 and barred the defendants from marketing this or any other product with unsupported claims.[26]

Unbelievably, Rose Creek (and other) Vitamin O products,
"oxygen" water coolers, and other oxygen scams remain available
online today making the same blatantly false claims about health
benefits that were supposedly prohibited by the FTC a decade ago.[27]
Websites still thumb their nose at the FTC and advertise "Vitamin
O Oxygen Therapy is a liquid taken sublingually or in water to help
oxygenate the body, which may benefit asthma, emphysema, fatigue,
candidiasis, immune suppressive diseases, brain and memory function, and heart problems."[28]

Bottled Water Weight-Loss Scams

Okay, most of us are fatter than we'd like. But eating less and exercising more just seems like, well, too much work. Surely there is an
easier way to lose weight. It turns out that there are lots of simple
ways to lose weight, marketers tell us. Unfortunately, most of them
are expensive frauds. Diet scams are as American as apple pie, with
the vanilla ice cream. Why not bottled water diet scams as well?

Excessive weight-loss claims for all sorts of products are common in the United States and some ineffective efforts have been
made to crack down on the worst offenders over the years. The FTC
rules for diet claims are similar to those for false advertising in general: an ad must be truthful and not misleading; and before disseminating an ad, advertisers must have adequate substantiation that

supports all objective claims. Given the prevalence of misleading dietary claims, the FTC has issued a broad ruling that claims of weight loss without extra physical activity or consuming fewer calories are inherently deceptive. As the FTC puts it: "These types of claims are simply inconsistent with existing scientific knowledge." Unfortunately, enforcement actions against the growing number of such claims in the United States are infrequent.[29] Through May 2003 the FTC has filed fewer than 200 cases of deceptive weight-loss advertising since the 1920s and not one involved misleading bottled water claims.[30]

The lack of enforcement has encouraged the proliferation of a whole panoply of "weight-loss" waters, such as "Skinny Water," "Jana Skinny Water," "Coolwater Trim," "Formas Luso" from Portugal, which states on its website: "*comprovado cientificamente, reduz o apetite*" (translation? "proven scientifically, it reduces the appetite"[31]), and eVamor Artesian Water, which wildly claims, among many other benefits, to reduce body fat.[32] Someone who drinks a lot of bottled water, or tap water for that matter, may indeed lose weight simply by suppressing appetite and eating less. But this benefit has nothing to do with any special properties conferred by the water itself as claimed by a variety of bottled waters, nor does it justify the exorbitant prices charged for these bottles.

In 2005 a company called Jana Water started marketing Jana Skinny Water, "a no-calorie water, enhanced with a unique combination of ingredients to help people lose and maintain their weight."[33] "Curbs appetite; increases fat burning," claims the version of the website posted in July 2005 and online through 2006. Those marketing the dietary power of the water argued that it could reduce appetite, increase metabolism, and block carbohydrate absorption if you drink enough of it, right before you eat. It can even "keep you good looking." To be sure, these weight-loss waters can slim down your bank account. Jana Skinny Water cost around $40 a case. In 2005 Jana Skinny Water won the award for "worst claim" in the Quackery and Fraud categories of the annual Slim Chance

Awards for Worst Diet Promotions. These awards are presented annually by the Healthy Weight Network and the National Council Against Health Fraud as part of their effort to counter widespread fraud in the weight-loss industry and "the exploitation by con artists of the public's seemingly insatiable desire to lose weight."[34]

What is the magic? For many "diet" waters, including Jana, the secret ingredient is hydroxycitric acid. What does this stuff do? "Current research on humans does not seem to indicate that hydroxycitric acid, the key component in G. cambogia [a plant found in Southeast Asia], has any effect on obesity," said Dr. Susan Bowerman, former assistant director of the University of California, Los Angeles Center for Human Nutrition, and a registered dietician and author.[35] A 2004 study in the American Journal of Clinical Nutrition concluded that hydroxycitric acid and a wide range of other dietary supplements could not be shown beyond a reasonable doubt to reduce weight.[36] They also concluded that "the evidence for most dietary supplements as aids in reducing body weight is not convincing." A 2005 review of twelve separate blind clinical trials of this stuff showed no consistent effect compared to placebos.[37] In the United Kingdom, in 2008, criticism from British regulators forced the producers of Skinny Water to concede that their claims are not supported by clinical studies.[38] The British Food Standards Agency warned the company that the product would violate new European Union laws against pseudoscientific claims. But these claims still abound throughout the bottled water industry, and U.S. regulators have yet to take action against weight-loss waters.[39]

Clustered and Magically Structured Waters

Perhaps the most common and weirdest bottled water claim is that water molecules can be magnetically, or electrically, or otherwise magically rearranged to promote health, energy, or flavor. Dozens of hucksters offer magically restructured waters, using pseudo-scientific language, doctored or misleading photos of ice crystals, and personal testimonials, often based on the bizarre writings of a

Dr. Masaru Emoto. Dr. Emoto (his doctorate is apparently in International Relations) claims that music, words, and thoughts combined with magic machines can affect the shape of frozen water crystals.[40] His followers point to photographs of "water crystals" that Emoto claims were affected by exposure to different things—beautiful crystals come from being exposed to classical music; ugly deformed crystals result from being exposed to heavy metal music. In fact, his followers say that if you just tape paper with written words on a water bottle, the water inside will restructure with different crystals: beautiful ones from words like "thank you" and "love and appreciation," and ugly ones from paper with things like "Adolph Hitler" or "you make me sick" written on them.[41] By the way, Emoto has also written that humans on Earth are descendants of criminal exiles from outer space—living in sort of an intergalactic Australia.[42]

Nineteenth-century German physicist Ludwig Friedrich Kämtz once wrote, "*Die Elektricität und der Magnetismus sind diejenigen Naturkräfte, mit denen Leute, die nichts von der Elektricität und dem Magnetismus verstehen, Alles erklären können.*" (That is, "Electricity and magnetism are those forces of nature by which people who know nothing about electricity and magnetism can explain everything."[43]) The claims for Dr. Emoto's Hexagonal Indigo Water, which sells for more than $30 per 8-ounce bottle, give a flavor for this large group of bottled waters.

> Using a combination of scalarwave energy, laser light, inert noble gases and frequency-emitting crystalline ceramic oscillators, Dr. Emoto's Water is hexagonally structured and imprinted with specific frequencies which are designed to stimulate and encourage mental coherence, symmetry and balance the qualities necessary for optimal functioning in a complex world.[44]

This kind of description has been called "pure techno-claptrap" by scientific debunker James Randi, yet Emoto's followers and other "clustered water" proponents are actively selling a wide range of bottled waters, all of which use variations of these claims. For example, Royal Springs, a Texas water bottler, sells water at $50 a case, claiming: "Rhythm Structured H_2O™ has smaller water clusters which move more easily in and out of cells in our body and more effectively carry in nutrients and wash out waste. The result is improved hydration, which allows our body to naturally detoxify itself."[45]

Or H_2Om (get the pun? *oooommm*), "The World's first Vibrationally charged, Interactive water," which "promotes positive thinking and positive energy for people and the planet."[46] The website for H_2Om repeats Emoto's claims that "recent scientific research has proven that water is directly effected [sic] by the words, sounds, and thoughts it is exposed to."[47] Before the water is shipped, the employees "charge the water in the storage facility with sound and music with intent."[48] Or Aquamantra's claim that their "energy-enhanced" bottled water "infused with luck gives Oscar nominees the edge."[49] As their website says, they also rely on:

> the scientific work-studies of Dr. Masaru Emoto, who over the past nine years has proven, through the use of hyper-powerful microscopes, that words written on bottles can affect the water's molecular structure. . . .
>
> Dr. Masaru Emoto . . . showed us the basic principles of quantum mechanics theory, whereby the molecular structure of water was changed by a Zen Buddhist monk's thought. Based on this premise, Aquamantra uses the design on its labels to affect the molecular structure of California natural spring water to make it more refreshing and wholesome to drink.[50]

I couldn't make this stuff up. They go on to claim:

> Take a piece of scotch tape and write "I Hate You" on the water, leave it overnight, in the morning take a sip of your "hate" water then take a sip of your regular water. Email us your feedback . . . we're anxious to learn your findings. That is precisely how we created Aquamantra. The words actually

change the molecular structure of the water, and most definitely changes [sic] the flavor of the water to taste deliciously smooth. This flavor is almost indescribable, its [sic] full of energy and its [sic] fantastic.[51]

The list of magically restructured waters goes on and on: in New Zealand one finds Blue Water selling for £11 a liter, which "has negative memories removed and replaced with beneficial energy patterns."[52] Vibe Water is marketed as a way to "tune" the body with energy patterns that can be imprinted in the water.[53] H₂X Scalar Wave Activated Water is made with "state of the art Quantum Star Scalar Wave Generators, Tesla Coils, proprietary Orgone Technology, Radionics Equipment, proprietary Hypersonic Frequency Generator Equipment, and Hyperdimensional Sacred Geometry and unique imprinting frequencies."[54] This last stuff is sold as a "concentrate," just like Dr. Emoto's Hexagonal Indigo water or Vitamin O—just add a milliliter of it to a liter of tap water or spring water. They sell it for around $30 for 30 ml, which means it costs around $1000 a liter! For just $99 for three bottles, you can get "concentrated" Zunami water "raised to a high level of electromagnetic power through a proprietary process. It is designed to restructure water into hexagonally organized bio-molecular clusters, providing better intracellular water exchange."[55] A New York company called Vava has marketed water treated with "low-level electromagnetic frequencies that change the crystallisation of the water, bringing about a physiological response starting at the cellular level."[56]

The Special Case of Penta Water

One of the most persistent examples of the bottled-water scam of "restructured" or specially "clustered" water is Penta Water. My first hint that some bottled water producers were hoping to sell more than water came nearly than a decade ago, long before the current explosion of interest and sales. One of my staff at the Pacific Institute walked into my office with a bottle of something called

Penta Water and asked if I had ever heard of it. Her sister, it turned out, drank nothing but Penta Water, at over $60 a case, specially ordered from Southern California. What was special about Penta Water? First produced in the late 1990s by a southern California businessman, William Holloway, Penta also claimed to have "restructured" the water through "molecular redefinition" and a special "oxygenation treatment." Its producers claim it has been "shown through highly technical scientific testing (Raman spectroscopy) to have 30 percent smaller molecular water clusters," to have "a higher boiling point and higher viscosity than normal water," and so on.[57]

Sales of Penta expanded rapidly with the development of an aggressive online marketing effort. As each new claim of Penta water's astounding benefits went unchallenged by FTC or FDA regulators, the list quickly grew. By mid-2001 the company was claiming that

> Penta . . . has been reduced to its purest state in nature— smaller clusters of H_2O molecules. These smaller clusters move through your body more quickly than other water, penetrating your cell membranes more easily. This means Penta is absorbed into your system faster and more completely. When you drink Penta, you're drinking the essence of water. You get hydrated faster, more efficiently, and more completely than with any other water on earth.[58]

By early 2002 Penta's webpages were asserting that the water had "superior hydration capability" and was "one of the purest drinking waters available." For support, the producers offered links to obscure and opaque scientific studies about "aquaporins" and water flow in cells.[59] By May 2003, the claims started to get even more specific, grandiose, and bizarre:

> Penta can help improve athletic performance, reduce acid load inside cells, increase the time cells live in adverse circumstances, and even reduce chromosomal mutation rates! Penta can do all

these things because it's truly different. The individual water molecules in Penta are arranged into small, stable clusters that more effectively get into your cells.[60]

Penta's claims eventually provoked a response from scientists and even from scientific skeptic James Randi, though not from U.S. regulators. Randi became famous as a magician and escape artist, and he has devoted much of his life to the James Randi Educational Foundation, committed to identifying, revealing, and debunking pseudoscientific and paranormal claims. His foundation has famously offered a million-dollar prize to anyone who can "show, under proper observing conditions, evidence of any paranormal, supernatural, or occult power or event." Hundreds of tests of ESP, dowsing, psychic power, astrology, faith healing, and more have been conducted; not a single one has passed.

In 2001 Penta's allegations provoked Randi to describe them as "a pack of lies designed to swindle and cheat, to steal money, and to rob the consumer," and he challenged them to apply for his prize money, noting

the sellers of "Penta" know they're lying, they do it purposefully, and they know they can get away with it because of the incredible inertia of the Federal agencies that *should* be protecting us against such deception and thievery. Those agencies just can't do the job, and they bumble about endlessly while the public continues to pay through the nose.[61]

Randi's attention was particularly drawn to the assertion of superior hydration and the claim that "test seeds [grown with Penta Water] would germinate in half the time as the control seeds."[62] Unlike so many of the wild claims made by bottled water marketers, here was something that could be directly and easily tested. Randi proposed to Holloway and Penta Water a series of double-blind tests for both the claims of superior hydration and faster-growing seeds.

Initially, Penta and Holloway accepted his invitation. Holloway told Randi that he wanted to use his own instrument, a "Bio Imped-ance Analyser," to test how hydrated humans get drinking Penta. Randi agreed, saying that the instrument would simply have to identify correctly which type of water, Penta or non-Penta, was drunk by 37 out of 50 subjects. If it could pass this relatively easy test, Holloway and Penta would then be eligible for the million-dollar prize. At this point, Holloway blinked and withdrew from the experiment, sending off a set of nasty emails that are still online at Randi's website.[63]

In late 2004 Penta Water's statements were more officially challenged in front of British regulators the Advertising Standards Authority (ASA) of the United Kingdom. Among the assertions that were challenged were statements made on a brochure distrib-uted by mail in England and on their webpage: "Proven faster, bet-ter hydration," "no ordinary water," "ultra-purified, restructured 'micro-water,'" "smaller stable clusters," "improves the environ-ment within your cells," "unique patented structure," and "unpar-alleled purity." The complainants challenged Penta on the grounds that their advertising misleadingly implied the product had health benefits over and above those of ordinary water and was "restructured."

Penta Water filed papers that they argued showed evidence of restructuring, and also several works in preparation that they claimed showed increased performance and recovery levels after exer-cise with Penta when compared with ordinary water. They also argued that, because Penta could (they claimed) hydrate more effi-ciently than tap water, it was better for health.

After independent review, the ASA concluded in March 2005 that the scientific evidence submitted completely failed to prove that Penta had any health benefits over and above those of ordinary water or had been "restructured" any differently from ordinary water to form stable smaller clusters. The ASA told Penta Water "not to repeat claims that implied the product was chemically unique, had been restructured or molecularly redesigned, or hydrated cells and improved physical performance better than tap water."[64]

Despite this ruling, Penta and its offspring such as Aqua-Rx water continue to make a wide range of health claims. As of 2007 the company's website claimed that Penta Water could dissolve "calcium oxalate monohydrate (the main substance in 85% of kidney stones) three times faster than normal water." It promoted "an increase in cell survivability by 266%." It claimed to lower "DNA chromosomal mutation rates" in human cells, and offered references to drinkers looking and feeling "more youthful, energetic, and all around better."[65] In 2008 and 2009 versions of their website claimed improved anti-oxidant activity, aid in weight loss, improved physical performance, faster hydration, increased muscle power and nerve firing, faster dissolving of kidney stones, increased cell survivability, and more, all without independent peer-reviewed scientific publications showing that drinking Penta water actually conveys any such benefits.[66] A footnote on the Penta website says "These statements have not been evaluated by the Food and Drug Administration."[67] Indeed. Why not, one wonders?

All of these various extreme claims use seemingly scientific language to convince an unsuspecting or uninformed public to spend money on things they don't need, and they prey on our fears that the alternative—in this case tap water—is unsafe. Scientists understand the physical and chemical properties of water. We know how to keep it clean, treat it to remove impurities, and process it for human consumption. But as long as charlatans see a way to capitalize on our ignorance or fear, and as long as our regulatory agencies keep their heads in the sand, snake-oil salesmen will always be with us. It is long past time for regulators to step in to protect the public from twenty-first-century snake-oil salesmen.

CHAPTER 9

Drinking Bottled Water: Sin or Salvation?

> If you are a sinner or evil in nature, this product may cause burning, intense heat, sweating, skin irritation, rashes, itchiness, vomiting, bloodshot and watery eyes, pale skin color, and oral irritations. Warning: Consuming Holy Drinking Water™ should not replace attending church or any other establishment of worship.
> — Warning label on the bottle and website of the company selling Holy Drinking Water

> By many measures, bottled water is a scam. . . . It's no wonder that some people even think it's a sin.
> — From the newsletter of the Fifth Episcopal District Women's Missionary Society of the African Methodist Episcopal Church[1]

WATER HAS LONG played a central role in religion and faith, rites of baptism, purification rituals, Sumerian, Hindu, Christian, and other myths and legends of deities using water to mete out punishment or blessings, and in the centrality of water to the sacredness of life. The use of water for spiritual cleansing is common to several religions including Judaism, Christianity, Hinduism, and Sikhism; but only the Catholic Church uses holy water as a sacramental to ward off evil. In the Catholic Church, water can be blessed by a priest or bishop and used for baptisms, blessings, consecration of a church, or aspersions during Mass. Only recently, however, have individuals explored the idea of commercializing different forms of "holy water."

Religion has also, of course, been used for decidedly unholy purposes. In a remarkable moment of transparency, sci-fi writer L. Ron Hubbard reportedly said, "If you want to make a little money, write a book. If you want to make a lot of money, create a religion." Hubbard took his own advice and did both: his 1950 self-help book, *Dianetics*, created a new religion—Scientology. Some water bottlers have taken note. Given all of the diverse and sophisticated efforts underway to get people to buy bottled water, it was only a small step to take for some bottled water producers to use religion as a marketing tool. Some of these efforts have been tongue-in-cheek; others have been completely serious. And for a third group, it is sometimes hard to tell.

One of the strangest bottled water products is Kabbalah Water, which combines bizarre claims like Dr. Emoto's molecular restructuring with unproven health assertions, religious mysticism, and a dash of pop culture. What is Kabbalah? The Kabbalah Centre in Los Angeles describes it like this:

> Kabbalah—the world's oldest body of spiritual wisdom—contains the long-hidden keys to the secrets of the universe as well as the keys to the mysteries of the human heart and soul. . . . Kabbalah shows in detail, how to navigate that vast terrain in order to remove every form of chaos, pain, and suffering. . . . Its purpose is to bring clarity, understanding, and freedom to our lives—and ultimately to erase even death itself.[2]

Others describe Kabbalah as a splinter cult with connections to an old strain of Jewish mysticism. Rabbi Immanuel Schochet, a Toronto-based expert on Jewish philosophy and mysticism, described the Kabbalah Centre in 2004 as "not just a cult, but a dangerous cult. They are distorting kabbalah . . . taking some of our sacred books and reducing it to mumbo jumbo, all kinds of hocus-pocus."[3] Rabbi David Wolpe of L.A.'s Conservative Sinai Temple was similarly critical: "Simple answers don't grow souls. Red threads and magic bottles of water don't change the world and don't change people. To the extent that deep spiritual truths are put in a blender and served as superficial pabulum—it's a disservice to a great tradition, and it is no better than spiritual snake oil."[4]

Rabbi Wolpe's comments about red threads and bottled water refer to another aspect of Kabbalah—their strong bent toward commercialism. Like most similar enterprises, Kabbalah supports itself with money from its followers and from the sales of, well, magical things, like red string that "protects us from the influences of the Evil Eye" ($26 for a package of string), scented candles whose "exact ingredients and preparation were directed by God to Moses" ($72 for a set), and most famously, Kabbalah water in bottles and in the form of a spray that uses "Kabbalistic technology" to "activate the cleansing power of water" ($10 for a small spray bottle). After all, if Kabbalah can "erase even death itself," people are going to be willing to pay a pretty penny for that.

One of the most famous and public followers of Kabbalah is pop icon Madonna and she made Kabbalah water famous, though she's jumped around in her bottled water devotions over the years. (Older fans will clearly remember a certain notorious incident with an Evian bottle.) I've always liked Madonna. Her music can be innovative; her efforts to push the limits of pop culture have been fun to watch, even when (or especially when) she steps over the line of cultural sensitivities, and some of her charity work has been laudable. But her ties with Kabbalah and her apparent willingness to not only swallow, but actively promote, their pricey and mystically infused bottled water are hard to abide. It would be a small thing if Madonna simply used Kabbalah water herself—she can certainly afford its high cost. It is quite another thing for her to promote Kabbalah water to her adoring fans and to link it to her charity work. According to the *San Francisco Chronicle*, during her 2006 tour Madonna brought in thousands of liters of Kabbalah water and required her dancers and crew to drink the water because she believes it has regenerative powers, a claim promoted by the Kabbalah Centre itself. "We charge the water with positive energy so that it has healing powers." In 2006 Reuters reported that her efforts to support a center for orphans in Malawi included requiring that they teach a curriculum linked to Kabbalah.

The best way to describe the claims made for Kabbalah Water is to share the mumbo-jumbo used by the Kabbalists themselves. Yehuda Berg, the son of the Los Angeles Kabbalah Centre's founder, asserts that the water is a tradition dating back centuries.[5] This is a particularly odd contention, since the actual claims made on behalf of the water seem to originate in the recent pseudoscientific claims of none other than Dr. Masaru Emoto, described earlier in this book. What follows is the description of Kabbalah water from the website kabbalahwater.com:

> Just as the sharing energy of water was fundamentally changed by human consciousness at the time of Noah's Flood, Kabbalah teaches that the power of consciousness can also reverse the change. . . .
>
> A truly sharing consciousness, channeled through certain Kabbalistic blessings and meditations, has the power to return water to its primordial state of completely positive, healing energy. Through the power of these meditations and the consciousness of sharing that is their foundation, Kabbalah Water came into being—and its miraculous powers of restoration and healing became available to the world. Infused with sharing consciousness, Kabbalah Water manifests water's primordial capacity to heal and protect. . . .
>
> The Kabbalistic blessings and meditations that are used to create Kabbalah Water, for example, bring about elegant and balanced crystalline structures in water, while negative consciousness has an opposite effect. . . . Because of its unique crystalline structure and fractal design, Kabbalah water is an excellent information transmitter. Positive, health-giving information is defined by symmetry and high energy, while low energy

and entropy—like static in TV or radio reception—characterize muddled information. Therefore, the condition of the water we take into our bodies determines the quality of the information being transmitted to our immune system, digestive system, circulatory system, and even to every atom of our bodies. . . .

The essence and foundation of Kabbalah Water is the consciousness of sharing which infuses it. Once, all the waters of the world were imbued with this consciousness. To learn more about the connection between consciousness and water, visit . . . [6]

And here the reader is directed to another website that uses the photographs of Dr. Emoto's water crystals, where, perhaps to no one's surprise, you can purchase a large variety of expensive water-related products.[7]

In mid-2005 another pop-music star, Britney Spears, jumped on the Kabbalah bandwagon, perhaps because of the influence of Madonna. (Her former flame Justin Timberlake had euphoniously described Spears as a "Madonna wannabe.") Celebrity observers reported that her enthusiasm for Kabbalah water was so intense that the pregnant Britney planned to "deliver her baby in a special pool filled with 1,000 one-liter bottles of specially blessed Kabbalah water" at a cost of nearly four thousand dollars.[8] Alas, celebrity births rarely go according to plan, and in the event the Spears-Federline offspring was delivered by more-traditional cesarean section at Santa Monica UCLA Medical Center.[9]

Okay, so what? In general, my tolerance for pseudoscientific nonsense is directly proportional to how harmless it is. If Britney wants to deliver her baby in a pool of Kabbalah water, who am I to complain—so long as her doctors have no complaints? And if Madonna drinks nothing else? Fine—it's probably better than what most pop stars are consuming. But my hackles start to rise when pseudoscience begins to crowd out real science in a way that threatens public health or the environment. In the case of Kabbalah water, their mystical claims have spilled out into the real world.

Enter Katherine Harris and Florida's environmental politics. Yes, that Katherine Harris. George W. Bush's Katherine Harris. In 2005 the *Orlando Sentinel* reported that the State of Florida had, at the "behest of then-Secretary of State Katherine Harris," studied the use of Kabbalah-blessed water as a cure for the very serious problem of citrus canker, a blight that was decimating Florida's vital agricultural sector. Researchers apparently were asked to test the ability of "Celestial Drops" to stop citrus canker. Celestial Drops is a magic potion with "improved fractal design," "infinite levels of order," and "high energy"—claims virtually identical to those made for Kabbalah water. Celestial Drops was promoted to Harris and Florida by Rabbi Abe Hardoon, a teacher of Kabbalah, and New York cardiologist Artur Spokojny, who said, "We have reversed entropy and reversed the second law of thermodynamics."[10] When asked by a Florida reporter if the canker project was related to Kabbalah, Hardoon replied, "It is, and it isn't," and he referred all further questions to the Kabbalah Centre of Los Angeles.[11] Oh, and by the way, the stuff didn't work on citrus canker.

Followers of Kabbalah are not the only ones using religion to sell bottled water. In recent years, more and more brands of bottled water have appeared on the market using religion as a marketing tool. And in the face of a growing backlash against bottled water, other religious communities are beginning to weigh in with moral and ethical judgments. Is drinking bottled water a path to salvation or damnation?

Those so inclined can now buy several versions of "holy" bottled water. One example is Holy Drinking Water, packaged at a private bottling plant in the city of Stockton, California. Businessman Brian Germann convinced clergy from the local Catholic and Anglican churches to pronounce blessings over his water, which he then labels and sells. Why would someone buy Holy Drinking Water at around $20 a case? To purify and protect your soul, apparently. "What if you could drink holy water as a defense against evil?" Germann said. As he explained to me, Germann hopes to get additional religious leaders to add their blessings and boost sales. Why? He's agnostic on the question of whether Jews or Protestants would get the full benefit of bottled water blessed only by Catholic or Anglican priests, and so he wants to expand the options available to the public.

Germann may have trouble getting a rabbi to produce a Jewish version. According to Judaism, food and water can be blessed before consumption by any member of the faith, but "I can't bless the water for someone else," said Rabbi Avrohom Brod of the Chabad of Stockton.[12] Similarly, Virginia Meagher, liturgy coordinator at the Catholic Diocese of Stockton, said bottled holy water isn't sacrilegious, but with notable restraint said, "It's probably not something we would encourage." Water, she said, can be blessed by a priest or deacon at any time, but it's then to be used to bless a new house or a sick person or in a religious ritual. Selling holy water, Meagher said, "seems to be against the reason we bless water."

Germann's bottles carry a label that warns sinners who drink the water that they may experience burning, intense heat, sweating, and skin irritations. This led to some amused commentary in the media, but Germann is keeping a straight face. The warning was intended "to be very serious," he told me. There have been no reported cases of adverse reactions among local sinners. One possible reason is that Holy Drinking Water is purifying souls. Another is that sinners are staying away from the stuff, preferring the less-risky secular brands. A third possibility, of course, is that Holy Drinking Water is, well, just water. Germann, whose main line of business is producing software for law-enforcement services, says he hopes to expand his operations to include a holy spring water version and sales of larger five-gallon coolers for home and office use.

In a more tongue-in-cheek vein comes Holy Spring Water sold out of Pennsylvania. "If you drink our water," the advertising for Holy Spring Water proclaims, "we guarantee that you will NOT GO TO HELL. If it tastes the same, costs the same, and may keep you out of hell, why (the hell) wouldn't you try it?" The sellers of Holy Spring Water even offer details on their website for how to

wash away specific sins. Lust, pride, and greed only require one bottle per transgression. Gluttony and anger require three bottles. Sloth
requires nine, perhaps because after nine bottles you have no choice
but to haul yourself out of the couch and head for the bathroom to
do penance.[13]

Another version of bottled water that relies on religious, albeit
tongue-in-cheek, messages is Liquid Salvation, offering "pure water
for an impure world" with a marketing image of a 1940s-style pin-up
girl portrayed as both a sexy angel and a seductive devil. The company is located in Henderson, Nevada, and sells a case of bottles for
$29.17 plus shipping. But this product goes beyond tongue-in-cheek
claims of salvation by claiming better hydration and, yes, a special
"patented" process that breaks apart "clustered" water molecules.
Miraculous indeed.[14]

There are many translations and interpretations of God's com-
mandments, depending on whether you're a follower of the Old Testament, the New Testament, the Qu'ran, or any of the other versions
of God's laws. I'm pretty sure that none of them explicitly says,
"Thou Shalt Not Drink Bottled Water." In fact, at the risk of being
struck by lightning, I imagine that there were times in the forty-year
wandering of the Jews through the desert that even Moses might have
found a vending machine with ice-cold bottled water (perhaps
Mayanot Eden or Neviot-Tevaa Hagalil brands?) to be a blessing.

In a far more serious vein, the growing revolt against bottled
water also has a religious component to it. Clean drinking water, like
air, some religious leaders argue, is a God-given resource that
shouldn't be packaged and sold. Others have gone further and
declared that drinking bottled water is immoral and even a sin. In
June 2005 a group called Presbyterians for Restoring Creation
(PRC) organized a conference called *Sharing the Waters of Life* at
which church members were asked to avoid bottled water, especially
those packaged in disposable PET containers. In May 2006 PRC
launched a campaign urging people to sign a pledge against bottled
water and to take the message to their churches.

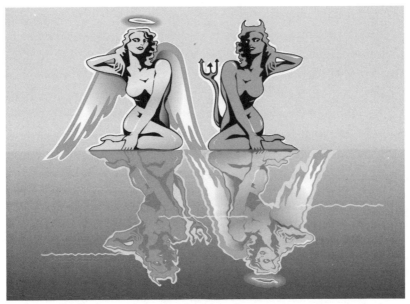

Liquid Salvation's "Pure water for an impure world." (Used with permission.)

In August 2006 the Thirty-Ninth General Council of the United Church of Canada (UCC) issued an advisory: "Avoid those purchased water bottles—where possible." The Council voted to discourage the purchase of bottled water by its congregations, noting its conviction that "water is a sacred gift" and "the privatization of water must be avoided." Together with the National Council of Churches (NCC), the UCC produced a documentary on the moral and ethical dangers of water privatization, including bottling water for sale in poor areas of the world. Cassandra Carmichael of the NCC said, "The moral call for us is not to privatize water. Water should be free for all."[15]

The following month, the Emmitsburg Province of Daughters of Charity adopted a formal stance against the use of bottled water and developed an educational program to help make the public aware of their concerns about the privatization of water. The Daughters of Charity belong to an international community of Catholic women consecrated by private vows to follow the teachings and inspiration of Vincent de Paul and to serve the poor. In their belief, commercial bottled water is one more barrier to serving the poor with access to the most basic of God's gifts: clean fresh water.

A few weeks after the adoption of this position, the National Coalition of American Nuns published an "Open Letter to Catholic Voters" calling for action in opposition to "the present bottled water culture promoted by the marketing agents of corporations such as Suez, Nestlé, and Coca-Cola." The Coalition's Board then committed not to buy commercially bottled water "unless absolute necessity requires such a purchase" and urged others to join in this effort.[16] In December 2006 Sister Mary Ann Coyle, who regards drinking bottled water as a sin, told the Religious News Service, "Our faith tells us to be just and not exploit the poor."[17] In 2009 twelve Episcopal bishops from the western United States issued a letter to members in advance of the church's annual General Convention in Anaheim, California. Their message? Stay away from bottled water, and don't bring it into the convention: "We urge you to encourage delegates not to buy bottled water, but instead to bring metal or ceramic water bottles that can be refilled with tap water."[18]

But religious doctrine can be an ambiguous thing, apparently even to the religious. Father Robert Sirico, a Roman Catholic priest and president of the Acton Institute, which promotes a more libertarian and market-oriented approach to religion, disputes that there is any moral problem with bottled water. "Where is the moral peril?" Father Sirico asked. To the bottled water consumer, he writes in an essay in the *National Catholic Register*: "You are not engaged in a sinful act. You are exercising a choice that is a human right, and supporting an ingenious institution—the free and enterprising economy—which is a powerful means of material liberation for the whole world."[19] I'm not sure what religion actually espouses the dogma of "material liberation" (not counting the religion of free-market capitalism, of course) or where consumer "choice" is codified in human rights law, but Father Sirico goes further, describing efforts to ban bottled water as "water socialism" and calling for the commodification of water as a necessary precondition for making water available to the masses. In other words, the failure to meet basic human needs for water is not the result of the failure of governments to provide safe water; it is the fault of "trade barriers and socialist structures." Water, Father Sirico says, should be treated like any other marketable product or simple commodity.

But is it? Water is not just another marketable product. It stirs far deeper feelings than the sales of carbonated soft drinks or blue jeans. And it is stimulating a far deeper response from local communities, environmental activists, and the general public, producing what may be a serious and permanent change in perception and hints at new thinking about both bottled water and water in general.

CHAPTER 10

Revolt: The Growing Campaign Against Bottled Water

I have no evidence to suggest it [the anti–bottled water campaign] has caused any decrease in sales. I think time will tell, but my sense of it is, it won't.
— Joe Doss, President of the International Bottled
Water Association (August 2007)[1]

As I described earlier, when I visited Google headquarters for a meeting in 2007, everyone was carrying around bottled water, offered free to all employees in coolers distributed in all the company's buildings. When I returned in 2009, those bottles were gone. A vigorous debate by the employees themselves had led to the elimination of that perk, and the employees, still carrying their laptops from meeting to meeting, were now carrying refillable plastic, aluminum, and steel water bottles. The war on bottled water has begun and the cachet of bottled water is slowly being replaced with embarrassment and discomfort.

More and more, the media is reporting on the problems and concerns with bottled water. After a colleague and I produced an analysis of the energy implications of bottled water, my phone at the Pacific Institute started ringing off the hook with calls from reporters, TV and radio shows, activists, local community groups, and concerned citizens, all wanting to know what to do about bottled water. What are the real impacts of bottled water? How much do we really use? What happens to the plastic? Who is really controlling the industry? What are the energy and greenhouse gas implications of bottling and moving large volumes of water? How can a small town find information and resources to fight off multinational corporations that want to build new bottling plants tapping local water supplies? Some of the many headlines tell the story:

- "San Francisco bans municipal purchases of bottled water."
- "Famous restaurateur Alice Waters bans commercial bottled water in her restaurant, Chez Panisse. Nestlé loses sales as Alice Waters bans bottled water."
- "Canada: Time to Turn Back to the Tap?"
- "Local communities oppose new bottling plants in California, Michigan, Maine."
- "New York City launches an ad campaign to support its own tap water. So does Paris."
- "The Mayor of Salt Lake City opposes city purchases of bottled water."
- "Corporate Accountability International launches a national anti–bottled water campaign."
- "The International Bottled Water Association moves to a crisis footing."

Some see ethical and moral reasons to fight bottled water. Some decry corporate control of such a precious and fundamentally public resource. Others reject bottled water for its economic and financial costs to the poor. Many are concerned about the environmental implications for the planet. Whatever the reason, a wide and growing range of individuals and groups—from cities, consumer groups, and environmental activists to restaurant owners, the religious community, and even politicians—have started to act to reduce and even eliminate their bottled water purchases and to influence others to do the same. At the same time, local communities are increasing efforts to challenge the production of bottled water. These efforts are squeezing the industry at two ends—putting pressure on demand and drying up supply. Will they make a difference? They already are. Sales are slowing, and in some places even falling, for the first time since the modern bottled water industry began.

In hindsight, there were hints that there might be limits to inexorable growth of bottled water markets. Sales of bottled water peaked in 2005 in France—the largest bottled water market in the world—and actually fell 2.5 percent the following year, at a time when sales were expanding rapidly elsewhere. According to *Brandweek*, an industry publication, by late 2007 bottled water sales were beginning to evaporate in other markets and regions as concern and public opposition started to grow. Early in 2008 the bottled water industry was still confident, at least in their official statements, that the growing opposition wouldn't affect sales. In March, Nestlé, which was already seeing a slowing in the growth of sales, tried to attribute it to "cooler weather."[2] In April, the Canadian Bottled Water Association stated "we are not seeing a decline in sales" in response to some worrying projections.[3] The IBWA in the United States remained outwardly assured through 2008 that sales would continue to grow. But there were hints things were changing. A PepsiCo spokesman acknowledged in the fall of 2008 that "negative press" had limited the growth of sales of Aquafina to 6 percent in the third quarter—a substantial drop from previous multi-digit growth rates—but the company tried to assure investors that sales growth would continue.

This was wishful thinking. When numbers for 2008 were finally released, the industry realized its first overall decline since bottled water sales started to be reported decades earlier. The Beverage Marketing Corporation confirmed in spring 2009 that overall sales in the United States had turned negative. In 2009 Nestlé Waters acknowledged that bottled water sales fell 1.6 percent in 2008—the first time the company had seen a drop in overall sales. Another global beverage group, Canadean, described U.S. demand as "switched off" and is now forecasting annual growth of less than 1 percent for the next five years, a significant deterioration from the double-digit growth rates over the past decade.4 France's Groupe Danone SA announced that its 2008 profits shrank 69 percent, in part because of declining sales of Evian bottled water in France, Spain, Japan, and the United Kingdom.5 In March 2009 the *Independent* reported that 2008 restaurant sales of bottled water in the United Kingdom dropped 9 percent compared with 2007 and that an increasing number of people request tap water when they eat out.6 Profit margins in the industry also fell because higher energy prices during the year led to an increase in both the cost of plastic and transportation—which accounts for a large part of the cost of producing bottled water. The drop in sales led Nestlé to announce that it would cut investment in its bottled water division to save money. CEO Paul Bulcke described 2009 as a year of "stabilization" for the bottled water division and they launched new marketing efforts to boost sales.7

The industry has tried to pin the drop in sales on the economy. Tom Lauria, vice president of Communications for the IBWA said in April 2009, "There's plenty of evidence that this recession is taking its toll on all forms of consumer spending. But there's little if any measurable evidence that activists have had an impact upon bottled water sales."8 Conversely, anti–bottled water activists were quick to claim credit. "Across the country municipalities, universities, churches, restaurants and unions are kicking out the bottle and turning on the tap," said Richard Girard, a spokesman for the Polaris Institute, a Canadian anti–bottled water group.9

And indeed, bottled water *is* under attack. Cities are banning municipal purchases of bottled water and imposing taxes or other fees to recover costs associated with bottled water use. Local communities that are the sources of bottled water are fighting the impacts of existing bottling plants on local streams, groundwater wells, and ecosystems, as well as mobilizing to stop the construction of new plants. Environmental activists have plunged into the fight with national and even global initiatives, using arguments about science, information on the environmental impact of the bottled water industry, tools of guilt and moral suasion, and even browbeating.

Cities Fights Back

France is strongly associated in people's minds with bottled water and the French are some of the largest consumers, drinking as much as 35 gallons per person per year (more than 100 liters per person per year)—much more than the average American. Famous French brands such as Perrier, Evian, Badoit, Volvic, Vittel, and others are shipped around the world and regularly found on the tables of Parisian cafés. But like New York, Paris is also proud of its municipal drinking water. For centuries Paris has been served by water from Roman aqueducts, the Canal de l'Ourcq, local rivers, and groundwater aquifers. These systems bring potable water throughout the city—to Paris's famous Wallace fountains, for example.

It is thus no surprise that Paris has been on the front lines of the war between bottled water and tap water. After years of growing pressure from bottled water, in 2005 the city launched a campaign to promote city tap water. They asked famous designer Pierre Cardin to create a glass carafe to be distributed to individuals and Parisian cafés to hold tap water. The city water agency produced 30,000 of the carafes and distributed them for free. In a marketing effort, the carafes were designed to fit in the door of home refrigerators and were marked with the Eiffel Tower and the Eau de Paris logo. "People buy bottled water because of the marketing, and we realized that if we were to win them back to the tap we would have to do some marketing of our own," said Franck Madureira of Eau de Paris.[10]

Some bottled water companies struck back, with new and aggressive advertising attacking Parisian tap water. "*Je ne bois pas l'eau que j'utilise*" ("I do not drink the water that I use"), declared a Parisian advertisement from Cristaline, a French mineral water, with an image of an open toilet with a red cross through it. Another Cristaline ad translates as "Nitrates, lead and chlorine . . . I don't save money on water I drink." The advertisements were published in defiance of a ruling from the national advertising standards agency, and so outraged Nelly Olin, the French environment minister, that she threatened legal actions: "I am angry. We do not accept that this company should cast aspersions on tap water. It is dishonest," she said.[11] In response to the ads, the President of Eau de Paris, the city water authority, arranged a blind water tasting at a café to show that consumers couldn't distinguish between tap water and Cristaline.

Paris isn't alone. New York City has always been proud of its water and it is one of only a handful of cities in the United States that wasn't required by the EPA to filter its source water, because it is so pure. Like Parisians, New Yorkers have begun to promote their tap water. In 2006 advertising artist David Droga, chairman of an avant-garde ad agency in New York called Droga5, produced a *pro bono* magazine campaign encouraging readers to drink tap water. The "tapproject.org," conducted in cooperation with UNICEF, produced articles and advertisements to encourage people to order tap water at participating restaurants, which then made a financial contribution to UN organizations working to provide safe water in developing countries.[12] In 2007 the city also committed $700,000 to promotional ads for the "Get Your Fill" campaign supporting local tap water. As part of the campaign, the city posted 1,400 subway and bus kiosk advertisements and paid for radio spots touting the tap.

The municipal responses against bottled water have not just come as a result of the desire to defend and support local tap water. In towns and cities around the world, expanding government purchases of bottled water for employees or city events has also become a big expense, and one that is increasingly viewed as an unnecessary luxury in a time of financial hardship. As money has grown tighter, so have city budgets, prompting elected officials to begin to question discretionary expenditures for a wide range of things, including bottled water. This is leading more and more municipalities to cancel purchases of bottled water for employees and city-sponsored events.

One of the first major cities to try to restrict bottled water use was Los Angeles all the way back in 1987, when Mayor Thomas Bradley issued an order restricting the use of city funds for purchasing bottled water. That order was increasingly ignored during the 1990s and early 2000s, but efforts to cut municipal bottled water use picked up steam again in the mid-2000s, when Los Angeles more formally banned city agencies from using city funds to buy bottled water. This wasn't a ban on bottled water in Los Angeles; rather Mayor Antonio Villaraigosa was explicit that "City employees who choose to buy bottled water in their office units at their own expense are encouraged to continue to do so. However, bottled water should not be provided at the city's expense."[13]

In 2006 the town Council in Rochdale, England, saved £6,500 by cutting back on biscuits at their meetings. That prompted a discussion of eliminating mineral water purchases in favor of serving local tap water and saving another £35,000. The Tory leader of the Council, Ashley Dearnley, said, "There is nothing wrong with tap water and the reality is we cannot afford to keep buying mineral water." In an unusual display of British bipartisanship, his Labour counterpart, Allen Brett, concurred, saying, "I think it is a good idea [to replace bottled water with tap water] and if Coun Dearnley hadn't proposed it, then it may have been suggested in the budget proposals."[14]

Also in 2006 Mayor Rocky Anderson of Salt Lake City sent a letter to his administrative heads requesting that they voluntarily stop serving bottled water at meetings, and in public statements he called bottled water "the greatest marketing scam of all time."[15] Mayor Anderson broadened his anti–bottled water campaign when he met with his colleagues at a meeting of the U.S. Conference of Mayors, an organization that represents mayors from over a thousand U.S. cities. At that meeting, Mayors Anderson, Gavin Newsom of San Francisco, and R. T. Rybak of Minneapolis sponsored a resolution underlining the importance of using municipal water and calling for studies on the environmental impacts of bottled water. The city of Seattle phased out bottled water sales for government offices in 2008, and Marty McOmber, spokesman for the mayor, summed up the issue when he said, "Seattle has one of the best municipal water supplies in the country. When you look at the cost of bottled water, both in terms of financial costs and costs on the environment, it's a pretty clear choice."[16]

The movement is spreading. Cities like San Francisco, Vancouver, St. Louis, Ann Arbor, Urbana, Santa Barbara, Manly, Toronto, Ottawa, Rome, Florence, Liverpool, and others, including larger and larger government entities, are moving to ban government purchases of bottled water and to endorse campaigns to promote local tap water. Toronto Mayor David Miller started requiring that tap water be made available at city council meetings and launched a campaign to "Fill with Toronto's High Quality Tap Water." In May 2009 San Mateo County, California, with a population of over 700,000 people, decided to stop buying bottled water with county funds. The county had been spending nearly $150,000 a year on bottled water, cups, and water coolers, and County Manager David Boesch asked the Board of Supervisors to pass an ordinance prohibiting the use of county funds for this purpose. As an alternative, the county will put in water filters and buy cups and pitchers so that tap water can be used. In anticipation of a common complaint about the taste of tap water, the county sponsored a taste test. More than half of the people participating couldn't tell the difference between Redwood City tap water and a local bottled water.[17]

As the financial crisis of 2008 and 2009 has hit budgets, even states are starting to look at saving money by reducing bottle water purchases. The Connecticut General Assembly found that the state spends at least $500,000 annually on bottled water and dispensers. Massachusetts spends about $600,000. Minnesota spent nearly $166,000 on bottled drinking water and water cooler/dispenser rentals, not including expenditures by large state institutions like the University of Minnesota, which spends another $180,000 annually.[18] All of these states are moving to cut these costs as they search for ways to save money. Bottled water now seems like a luxury, not a necessity.

Some local governments are using other tools to discourage use of bottled water or to recover the environmental costs associated with its use. Chicago has imposed a landmark tax of a nickel on each bottle of water sold in order to help defray the additional costs to the city of disposing of the plastic waste. The bottled water industry, including the IBWA, the American Beverage Association, and some Illinois merchant associations, promptly sued, fearing a tidal wave of new fees or taxes imposed on their product. In June 2009 the Cook County Circuit Court in Illinois ruled that Chicago's tax was legal. One of the most important arguments made by the city, and upheld by the court, was that the environmental impacts of bottled water "can generally be avoided in Chicago by drinking tap water, which is a readily available, inexpensive, safe, and environmentally friendly alternative."[19]

We are also seeing a modest revival of another approach to convince people to reduce purchases of bottled water—the restoration of the reputation and availability of the lowly water fountain. Modern water fountains are made without lead and they can both chill and filter the water. The Haws Corporation, founded in 1909 by a plumber from Berkeley, California, now sells a variety of models that include filters, coolers, variable stream heights, and more. Haws also offers a modern "hydration station" that can be used to fill portable water bottles. The Elkay Corporation in Illinois advertises fountains that include filters that remove viruses and cysts such as *Cryptosporidium* and *Giardia*, along with lead and chlorine. In a few airports, schools, parks, and other public spaces, new and highly visible state-of-the-art fountains are being installed. In January 2008 the Minneapolis City Council approved $500,000 for the construction of ten new public drinking fountains, each designed by a different Minnesota artist.[20] Community groups in New York are calling for the city to improve the condition of park fountains. In the summer of 2008 the Mayor of London, Boris Johnson, called for new water fountains to be put in parks and public spaces across the city, in part as an alternative to plastic bottled water. Said the mayor, "If this place is generally getting hotter and people are going off buying bottled water, I think we should have a new era of public fountains."[21] A recent study in German grade schools found that water fountains, combined with lesson plans about the benefits of drinking water, led to a drop in the number of overweight children, prompting calls for new school fountains.[22] The city council of Toronto voted in December 2008 to ban the sale and provision of bottled water in city facilities and to invest in fixing old water fountains and installing new ones. The Manly Council in Australia recently installed six high-tech water fountains on main streets and along the beach as part of a campaign against bottled water. In the fall of 2009 I received a phone call from a design firm working on the new terminal at San Francisco Airport, asking for information about global water issues to accompany the new "hydration stations" they were planning to put throughout the terminal. And the University of Central Florida's stadium now has fifty new water fountains.

Local Water

An increasing number of restaurants have also been in the front lines of the campaign against bottled water, despite the fact that bottled water can be a significant source of revenue. Restaurants know that they can boost profits, and servers can boost tips, by making water another commodity. Yet more and more restaurateurs are shifting to encourage healthy foods and sustainable agriculture grown nearby—a campaign many call "local food." Maybe it is time to launch a "local water" campaign as well to encourage consumers to turn away from bottled water and back toward local sources of supply.

In 2003 Larry Mindel opened Poggio, an upscale restaurant in Sausalito, California, across from San Francisco. From the beginning Mindel refused to push bottled water on his customers, instead serving filtered tap water and even sparkling tap water carbonated at the restaurant. He knows he could make more money if he and his servers pushed bottled water, but Mindel says it gives him a "stab" to charge for water. "Haven't you gone to a restaurant and they just expect you to order two or three bottles of water and it's $27 by the time you're done?" While some restaurants fear the loss of revenues, the environmental advantages were more important to Mindel. Many of his customers seem to agree. "I love that," said Joan Nitis. Her friend Anita Pira agreed, "We can buy more wine."[23]

Incanto, also in the San Francisco Bay Area, switched to serving only tap water in reusable carafes in the mid-2000s. "Serving our local water in reusable carafes makes more sense for the environment than manufacturing thousands of single-use glass bottles for someone to use once and throw away," says their website.[24] They have good reason to serve local tap water: San Francisco's water comes from a pristine watershed inside of Yosemite National Park in the Sierra Nevada.

Perhaps the highest profile restaurateur to ban bottled water is famed foodie Alice Waters, whose world-renowned Chez Panisse in my hometown of Berkeley, California, stopped offering commercial still waters in 2006 and ended sales of sparkling water in 2007 when they installed their own carbonator. "All this energy to bottle water, carbonate it, put it in the glass, ship it and truck it to our restaurant— it was such a waste," said Chez Panisse's general manager, Mike Kossa-Rienzi. The restaurant now provides free filtered or carbonated tap water, a move that received a huge amount of press attention when it was announced, adding momentum to the anti–bottled water movement.[25] Many more examples have been in the news. In New York City's Del Posto restaurant, chef Mario Batali and co-owner Joseph Bastianich removed bottled water from the menu in 2007. In Chapel Hill, North Carolina, chef Bret Jennings stopped serving bottled still water in his restaurant Elaine's in 2008.[26] These chefs and restaurant owners are unusual, not yet typical. But they are making high-profile public statements that have contributed to the perception that perhaps we can afford to rethink our bottled water purchases. The industry has responded—it decries the imposition of what it labels a "no choice policy"[27]—but the trend away from pushing bottled water in restaurants seems to be accelerating at the same time that local efforts to put limits on bottling plants are expanding.

Fighting Bottled Water at the Source

Serious opposition to bottled water has spread from the cities and towns where bottled water is consumed to the small communities where big and small bottlers produce it or where they want to build new factories to satisfy projected increases in demand. Local efforts to cash in on the bottled water phenomena have led to a growing number of confrontations as water resources that local residents have taken for granted have begun to disappear, streams have dried up, and groundwater levels have dropped when someone launches a local bottled water business. A number of these clashes have been chronicled in recent books and films, especially some of the major controversies around efforts by major companies like Nestlé in Michigan, California, Maine, and elsewhere.

One of the first blows against the bottling, export, and sale of local water came in the late 1990s in the small mountain community of Idyllwild in the San Jacinto Mountains, a couple of hours drive from the heart of Los Angeles. The town is small and peaceful, and the 3,500 inhabitants like it that way. The residents treasure their physical and mental distance from Los Angeles, and their biggest worry, besides the ever-present risk of forest fires, is the encroaching metropolis of Southern California. In the late 1990s a local resident, Chuck Stroud, began to notice that Lily Creek, a small stream he'd been visiting for many years, was drying up. And in mid-1998 he found out why. A local resident, Paul Black, had begun to pump groundwater from a well drilled on his land and to sell it as Idyllwild Mountain Spring Water. That groundwater had fed Lily Creek as well as aquatic habitat and trees that protected threatened desert species, which started to die off as water flows dropped. In the residential neighborhood around Black's property, water tanker trucks started to interfere with traffic on the small local roads.

Expressing the view common to most private sellers of water, Paul Black told a reporter from the *New York Times* in 2003, '"I see a very effective use of the water. It's safe, clean drinking water. Would you let it go, or would you do something with it?"'On the other side, Daniel Pietsch, an Idyllwild merchant who helped organize opposition to the bottled water operation said, "We're here because we have a lot of dying trees, and we don't like water going off our hill to be put in plastic bottles. We think it should be in our streams and our ground."[28]

In Idyllwild, things got so out of hand that neighbors filed civil complaints and organized public demonstrations. Tempers flared and cars of protesters, including a pickup truck owned by Pietsch, were vandalized. Paul Black tried to run over a protestor with his white Mercedes SUV and was arrested on charges of assault with a deadly weapon. A court found him guilty of a single count of battery, sentenced him to serve sixty days on consecutive weekends at the Larry Smith Correctional Facility in Banning, and ordered him to participate in an anger-management program. In January 2004 he was also ordered to pay $5,000 in restitution for damage to Pietsch's truck. Ultimately, environmental and land-use objections were effective with government agencies, and the waterworks was shut down.

The fight in Idyllwild will sound familiar to those who are fighting over bottled water today. Stroud's initial discovery of the bottled water withdrawals and the community's subsequent efforts to protect Lily Creek led to local activism, threats of violence, direct confrontations, and acts of vandalism.[29] At the heart of these fights is a fundamental difference in philosophy between those who see a free-flowing river or a pristine groundwater aquifer as a wasted resource begging to be exploited, and those who value resources left in place to provide for natural systems and aesthetic benefits or to satisfy local community needs.

Concerns about bottled water have been growing especially

rapidly in rural communities like Idyllwild, and Nestlé has been a high-profile target because of their strong demand for spring water, which must come from pristine, often rural, sources. In 2006 it was discovered that the Fujiaqua Company, a Nestlé affiliate in Japan, had been taking water for eight years from the Fujihakone Izu National Park without government permission.[30] In Crystal Springs, Florida, a major Nestlé bottling subsidiary—Zephyrhills—drew public protests when the company tried to increase local spring water withdrawals sixfold. Environmentalists there are fighting to block bottlers' operations and restrict the issuance of state permits in locales where companies can tap underground springs for minimal fees of a few hundred dollars a year. The state of Maine, where agencies have approved 15 bulk water exports and 18 bottled water facilities since 1987, has also seen more than its share of bottled water controversies.[31] In Freyburg, Maine, one of the towns where Nestlé produces water for its Poland Spring brand, residents have claimed the company is depleting the aquifer and they are fighting against expansion plans. A local organization, H$_2$O for ME, has challenged the state's Department of Health and Human Services for failing to enforce a 1987 state law that prohibits bulk transportation of water away from the source. As part of this effort, residents are trying to get the state to impose a per-gallon fee on "nontraditional" users.

Nestlé also ran into a buzzsaw of opposition in Northern California for their proposal to build a massive new spring water plant in the town of McCloud, near Mount Shasta. Compared to Paul Black's little bottling operation, the McCloud facility was a monster. As originally proposed, Nestlé planned to bottle a minimum of 500 million gallons of spring water each year from the McCloud River watershed, along with a potentially unlimited amount of groundwater from the same basin.[32] The initial 100-year contract signed with the town called for Nestlé to build a one million square-foot water-bottling facility on the site of the former CalCedar lumber mill. This is at least double the size of the huge Arrowhead plant in Cabazon that I visited, and one report estimated that this single cavernous building could contain every existing building in the community.33 The amount of water Nestlé wanted to bottle is about equal to the entire production of Nestlé's East Coast brand, Poland Spring.

Like most big industrial projects, this proposal had both supporters and opponents in the local community. Supporters saw benefits for the economically depressed town. Opponents worried that the proposed pumping would dry up local aquifers, deplete a major trout stream, and worsen truck traffic. Under the initial agreement, Nestlé would have paid the town of McCloud only $0.00008 for each gallon of water, or 8 cents per thousand gallons it took from McCloud's springs.34 A retailer would sell that same gallon of spring water in separate plastic bottles for as much as $5 or more. Even if Nestlé only received one fifth of the retail cost—a typical industry claim—the McCloud plant would have brought them over $500 million dollars a year. Big business indeed. Local opposition led Nestlé in August 2008 to announce they would renegotiate their contract and that they would reduce the size of the facility and annual water consumption. The opposition to the plant continued, however, and in September 2009, after six years of controversy, Nestlé withdrew its plans for a plant in McCloud.

In 2009 another proposal by Nestlé to draw 65 million gallons a year of spring water from along the Arkansas River in Colorado also ran into local opposition. The spring would be Nestlé's first in Colorado. Water would be pumped from groundwater wells by the river and trucked out of the basin to an Arrowhead bottling plant in Denver. At present Nestlé cannot satisfy the demand for their Arrowhead Spring water in Colorado without trucking water from other plants as far away as California. Press reports suggest that Nestlé has plans to tap springs in several other locations in Colorado as well. While a company spokesman said, "It's such a small—what I'll call a surgical—extraction of spring water from this aquifer," the permit asks for permission to withdraw 10 percent of the flow from these springs.35

Banning the Bottle: The Beginning of a Civil Movement

As the scope and intensity of the opposition to bottled water has expanded, so has the sophistication of the campaigns. One of the most organized efforts to move people away from the bottle is coming from the advocacy group Corporate Accountability International (CAI). CAI began in 1977 as Infact with a mission to wage "campaigns that challenge irresponsible and dangerous actions by corporate giants." Among their early campaigns were calls for reforms in the marketing of infant formula in poor countries and increased restrictions on international sales of tobacco.

For the past few years CAI has been running a campaign called "Think Outside the Bottle" to combat "aggressive attempts to turn water from a basic human right into an unaffordable luxury." They run an active media campaign, conduct highly public taste tests in big cities, and work with mayors and city managers to try to reduce or ban purchases of bottled water by public agencies. "Bottled water is bad for taxpayers, bad for public water systems, and bad for the environment," says Deborah Lapidus, a national organizer with CAI.[36] In Canada, a comparable effort called the "Back to the Tap" movement has been launched by university campuses, church groups, municipalities, and advocacy groups. In the United Kingdom, Friends of the Earth and the Food Commission, an independent watchdog on food issues, has called bottled water "environmental madness" and pushed for the public to stop buying it.[37]

Colleges and universities are also getting involved in anti-bottled water efforts. Students at Leeds University in England voted in 2008 to ban bottled water in bars, cafés, and shops on their campus—a decision that was heavily covered by the British press.[38] "Bottled water companies must fear that the days of fooling people into paying handsomely for a product they could get for free are numbered," said Sophie Haydock in a commentary in the *Guardian*.[39] Washington University in St. Louis, Missouri, banned the sale of bottled water on campus, and other U.S. schools, including Brandeis University, Penn State, and Ohio Wesleyan University, have begun moving toward similar bans. In Canada, the University of Winnipeg and Memorial University in Newfoundland have eliminated the sale of bottled water on their campuses, and in February 2009 students at McGill University voted to end the sale and distribution of bottled water within the Student Union building and to lobby the University administration to eliminate the sale and distribution of all bottled water on the campus.[40]

Bottled Water Companies Fight Back

The bottled water industry is fighting back. As anti–bottled water efforts accelerate and threaten sales and profits, the industry has begun to respond with a growing public relations push, increased spending on advertising, new lobbying efforts to stop legislation they don't like, and a general battening down of the PR hatches. The most coordinated effort to defend bottled water is coming from the International Bottled Water Association. The IBWA has dramatically ramped up its response to criticisms of bottled water. In 2006 IBWA wrote 14 letters to the editor or editorial comments and responded to 105 media interviews. In just the first nine months of 2007 they wrote 34 letters to the editor and responded to over 160 media interview requests.[41] In August 2007 the IBWA took out full-page ads in the *San Francisco Chronicle* and the *New York Times* responding to attacks on the industry. In 2008 they launched attacks on environmental groups, the U.S. Conference of Mayors, and publications critical of bottled water (as no doubt they will on this book as well). In 2009 they began releasing YouTube videos promoting bottled water safety and profiling small family-owned bottlers, and they filed lawsuits against what they see as bad laws or unfair business practices. The IBWA has also directly accused Corporate Accountability International of confusing customers and misleading the public, saying, "The CAI campaign is based on factual errors and subjective viewpoints on bottled water and does nothing more than confuse and misinform consumers."[42]

Other industry efforts are underway as well. In Great Britain, bottlers (including Nestlé, Danone, and Highland Spring) created a lobby group call the Natural Hydration Council to respond to opposition to bottled water. Jeremy Clarke, the director of the council, says the companies want to bring "hard facts" and "real science" to the debate. "Bottled water is the healthiest and greenest drink on the shelves," he said.[43] Some companies have stopped responding to media requests altogether, perhaps in the hopes that anti–bottled water campaigns will just dry up and blow away. When a reporter pursuing a bottled water story called Fiji Water in California in August 2007, he was told by a company representative, "We don't like talking to the media, whether it's positive, negative, or indifferent."[44]

The industry is also beginning to challenge municipal government efforts to promote local tap water, and one of the key battlegrounds is Florida, which ranks third behind Texas and California in bottled water purchases, consuming more than 575 million gallons a year. When Miami–Dade County, Florida, ran a series of radio advertisements between August and October 2008 touting the county's tap water as cheaper, safer, and purer than bottled water, the bottled water industry threatened to sue. Over a five-week period the county bought over 1,600 spots on 12 FM radio stations. The ads featured a talking water faucet: "You think bottled water is purer and safer? You think it's better? Well, you're wrong. It's just the opposite . . ." Although no specific bottled water brands were mentioned, Nestlé Waters North America, which operates several plants in Zephyrhills and Madison County and can draw nearly a billion gallons a year from four springs for sale throughout the southeastern United States, was particularly incensed. "It's an attack on the integrity of the company," said a Nestlé spokesman, "It's an attack on the product we produce."[45] A law firm representing Nestlé sent a letter to the county demanding they pull the ads, and the company also sent a complaint to the Florida attorney general. The *Miami Herald* newspaper reported that the International Bottled Water Association threatened "similar action," though the issue seems to have been dropped when the ads ended.

The bottled water industry has also launched their own new campaigns to promote and encourage bottled water use and to shoot down any efforts to restrict their operations. In New Mexico in 2007, a state senate bill to exempt bottled water from the state's gross receipts tax was approved after intense lobbying by bottlers. The state had earlier lifted the tax from most groceries and food staples but left it in place for things like coffee sold in cafés and for bottled water.[46] At the same time, bottlers continue to oppose efforts to add bottled water to bottle recycling bills, which were often put in place long before there was a substantial bottled water presence on grocery shelves or in our landfills. In 2009 Nestlé Waters North America sued New York State to block efforts to expand that state's bottle bill to include bottled water. Among other things, the measure expanded five-cent deposits from just carbonated beverages, wine coolers, and beer, to include bottled water.[47]

Bottlers have reason to be worried. The sales drop in 2008—the first ever reported—seems to represent a clear change in public perceptions about bottled water. While the bottled water companies, in public, believe that the drop can be attributed to the economic downturn, in private they must fear that the anti–bottled water campaigns are having an effect. Certainly, the environmental problems with bottled water, the economic costs to pocketbooks, and the growing support for improving tap water quality and reliability are all contributing to new thinking about the simple act of buying a plastic bottle of water. Bottled water is not likely to disappear, nor necessarily should it. But it is going to be increasingly difficult for the industry to argue that bottled water is just another benign commercial product, like soda, or soap, or blue jeans. There are going to have to be fundamental changes in the rules for licensing, bottling, and selling water; new more "ethical" or "green" alternatives, and far stronger government regulation and oversight to protect the public interest and health. The bottled water revolt is here, it is real, and it is not going away.

CHAPTER 11

Green Water?
The Effort to Produce
Ethical Bottled Water

I'm probably the only operator of a bottled water company who would
tell you that you should drink tap water—but if you're going to buy a
bottle of water, we want to provide an ethical option.
— Kori Chilibeck, founder of Earth Water[1]

Ethical bottled water must be the biggest oxymoron of our time.
— Michael Smith, *Green (Living) Review*

Is THERE A middle ground between an unconstrained bottled
water industry and a complete ban on the product, as some activists
would like? Some see such a middle ground in attempts to market
"ethical" brands of bottled water. Can bottled water be made "ethical?" Several entrepreneurs think so. Their efforts range from
attempts of the biggest bottlers to decrease the environmental consequences of their production to commitments on the part of some
bottlers to donate some or even all profits from sales to charitable
organizations, including those working to provide safe water and
sanitation to poor communities.

Because much of the energy and environmental costs of bottled
water are tied up in the plastic bottle, some major producers are
responding to the growing opposition to bottled water by making

changes in their operations and products. As we saw earlier, Nestlé, for example, is moving toward "lightweighting"—reducing the amount of plastic needed to make each bottle—and their newest bottling plants are being built to meet LEED Green Building Council standards. Nestlé recently introduced their "Eco-shape®" bottle, which reduces the weight of their standard PET bottle by around 30 percent. This effort was accompanied by a major publicity blitz; their website proclaims: "Easier to hold, easier to live with" and "A better bottle for you and our environment."[2] Both Coca-Cola and PepsiCo have also introduced lighter bottles, but their standard bottle is still substantially heavier than Nestlé's.

Coca-Cola and PepsiCo have both launched other efforts to address the water implications of some of their beverage activities around the world. Rather than focus on the specific impacts of their bottled water business, they have ramped up efforts to understand how their companies use or abuse water resources and to reduce the consequences of this water use in local communities, clean up or reduce their discharge of wastes into water systems, and improve the transparency of their operations. Coca-Cola, in particular, has moved aggressively to try to clean up their image and their operations after receiving bad publicity in India and elsewhere for their use of water in beverage production. For example, in 2007 they announced that they were going to focus on three aspects of their water impacts by working to improve their water-use efficiency, to treat all water to "a level that supports aquatic life and agriculture," and most controversially, to become "water neutral" in their overall operations, which they define as replacing the water that is consumed when making their products.[3] For example, the company is trying to figure out how to replace in rivers or groundwater the three or four liters of water that are consumed when they make a liter of carbonated soft drink, but they are not, at the moment, addressing the thousands of liters of water that may be required to grow the sugar or corn used in the same one-liter bottle of beverage. In February 2009 Coca-Cola also opened the world's largest PET bottle-to-bottle recycling plant in Spartanburg, North Carolina—one of the first serious U.S. efforts to boost the amount of recycled PET in beverage bottles.4

A panoply of smaller entrepreneurs sees the large market for bottled water as an opportunity to do something good for the planet. Rather than fiddling around the edges with lighter PET bottles, or improving the water efficiency of bottling plants, some are taking a different approach, looking to new models of production and operation. While it is hard to ascribe motives to these bottlers, most seem to feel that if people are going to buy bottled water, they might as well have the choice of contributing something positive. Most of these bottlers are committing a portion of their profits to good causes and exploring less environmentally damaging packaging options.

Perhaps the most significant attempt to build an ethical brand in bottled water involves Ethos Water—the brainchild of Peter Thum. Ethos was begun by Thum and his friend Jonathan Greenblatt in the classic style of business startups and is now part of the multinational corporation Starbucks. I first met the founders of Ethos in early 2005, after they had started the company and when they were seriously considering moving from a local model to national bottling and distribution. Thum and Greenblatt came to visit me at the Pacific Institute and we talked for several hours about bottled water, ethics, and the environment.

Thum grew up in the upper-middle-class, and, as he describes it, "unreal" surroundings of Southern California, giving little thought to water issues. He went to business school at the Kellogg School of Management at Northwestern University, where he roomed with Greenblatt, his future partner in Ethos Water. In the fall of 2000 Thum was working in England for the McKinsey consulting firm and was sent to South Africa for six months to help reposition the brand of a winery near Capetown. While there he was exposed to the water poverty that afflicts so many people in South Africa, and he became immersed in that country's intense water debates. There are few countries with more difficult and complex water problems, or more innovative efforts underway to solve them. As Thum told me, he came to realize that "without solving water and sanitation issues, efforts to address all other problems are like building a house on sand." On his return to England, he was assigned to another project to help a soda and bottled water manufacturer and realized there must be a way to create a beverage brand to take advantage of the fact that more and more consumers were looking for emotional benefits "beyond just satisfying their thirst or convenience."

By the summer of 2002 Thum had quit his job, written a business plan for Ethos, and moved to New York to pursue his idea for a bottled water company that would enable consumers of bottled water help address the world water crisis. The basic premise was that Ethos could capitalize on the growing market for bottled water as a tool for generating both the funds and the awareness necessary to help meet basic needs for water in developing countries. And this would also provide the brand its differentiation from all of the other waters on the market. By the end of that year, he recruited Greenblatt to join the Ethos effort. In late spring 2003 Thum moved to California where Greenblatt lived with his wife. Thum put together the pieces of the supply chain while Greenblatt worked to raise funds. Thum met with bottlers, found a producer who could make the appealing package they wanted, and selected a water supplier.

Ethos Water was born about 12 weeks after Thum moved to California. As a way to make the brand known, he and Greenblatt sought their first customers in places where celebrities hang out. The original obligation of Ethos was to give 50 percent of their profits to organizations supporting water and sanitation projects in developing countries, which they estimated would be around 1.9 cents per bottle over the projected life of the brand. Thum concluded that a few high-profile customers would help them to launch the brand, and so they introduced their product at the Fred Segel Café on Melrose Avenue in Los Angeles, which advertises "homemade pastas with a side of celebrity sightings." They quickly expanded to cafes and restaurants up and down high-end Los Angeles. By October 2003 Ethos sales were sufficiently encouraging to convince

Greenblatt to quit his job as an executive, work full time on Ethos, and search for outside angel funding to help them expand production. In February 2004 Ethos went as a corporate sponsor to the famous TED (Technology, Entertainment, and Design) conference, where they did what every entrepreneur should do—they schmoozed and pitched. And among the people they pitched were Pam and Pierre Omidyar, the founders of eBay and the philanthropic Omidyar Network.

The Omidyars liked the idea of an ethical bottled water brand and made an equity investment in Ethos that permitted them to grow further and, more important, to pursue Starbucks as an outlet. The thousands of Starbucks cafes and millions of customers could get them over the "scale hurdle" they faced, and in the summer of 2004 they met with Howard Schultz, the chairman and CEO of Starbucks. Schultz was also looking for a socially responsible way to sell bottled water and liked the Ethos brand better than the brand they were currently selling. By April 2005 Greenblatt and Thum had negotiated a deal: Starbucks would buy the fledgling company and sell the water in their stores, committing 5 cents for every bottle sold to nonprofits and agreeing to raise $10 million for water projects by 2010. Thum and Greenblatt took executive positions at Starbucks to help launch the expansion. By the end of 2008 Starbucks had made over $6 million in grant commitments that they claim will help over 420,000 people in Africa, Asia, and Latin America.

The idea of ethical bottled water is spreading. A Canadian company called Earth Water, which began operations in 2004, claims to donate 100 percent of net profits to water programs in developing countries and in 2007 introduced a corn-based biodegradable bottle; the company also works directly with the United Nations High Commissioner for Refugees (UNHCR). Reflecting the apparent contradiction between bottled water and ethical consumerism, Earth Water's CEO and founder, Kori Chilibeck, noted in August 2007, "This is not a cure-all solution, but we know that if other bottlers follow our lead, it will have a huge impact."5

Examples of "Ethical" Bottled Water

Frank Water, United Kingdom: Frank Water is a water charity that supports sustainable clean water projects in developing countries. Created by award-winning social entrepreneur, Katie Alcott, Frank Water says it gives 100 percent of its profits to charity. http://www.frankwater.com/.

One Water and Global Ethics, United Kingdom: In 2005 British entrepreneur Duncan Goose created One Water and Global Ethics, which return all net profits on their bottled water to irrigation and drinking water projects in developing countries, a joint undertaking with PlayPumps International. In 2009 One Water expanded into the United States and Australia. http://www.onedifference.org/water.

Belu Spring Water, United Kingdom: Belu was founded by Reed Paget and colleagues and donates 100 percent of net profits to WaterAid, which distributes it to clean-water projects across Africa and Asia. They also claim to be the United Kingdom's first carbon-neutral bottled water. The water is available at festivals, some London restaurants, and the Tesco and Waitrose supermarket chains in the U.K. http://www.belu.org/.

Aquaid Ltd., United Kingdom: This company reportedly donates 10 percent of rental income from its water coolers and 35p for every 12- or 19-liter bottle of water sold to various water-development projects in Malawi through Christian Aid and Pump Aid. http://www.aquaid.co.uk/.

continued

In Great Britain, a socially conscious businessman, Reed Paget, set up a company that uses glass and corn-based biodegradable bottles to package Shropshire spring water from northwestern England. The product—Belu Natural Mineral Water—was first marketed in 2004. Paget's website says that 100 percent of the profits go to water projects in developing countries, with their first project in Tamil Nadu, India. In 2008 they claimed to be the United Kingdom's first "carbon-neutral bottled water."[6]

Another Englishman, Duncan Goose, founded a nonprofit corporation called Global Ethics and a bottled water company called One Water, which returns all net profits to irrigation and drinking water projects in developing countries. Goose was born and raised in Edinburgh and worked for several years in marketing and consulting before making money selling a firm he helped create. With the profits

Examples of "Ethical" Bottled Water, *continued*

Ethos Water, United States: The sale of a bottle of Ethos water at a Starbucks outlet leads to the contribution of 5 cents to water-supply and sanitation projects in developing countries. Starbucks has set a goal of providing at least $10 million by 2010 for such projects. http://www.ethoswater.com/.

Earth Water International, Canada: Earth Water International's mandate is to give 100 percent of net profits to the UNHCR (the United Nations Refugee Agency) to provide clean drinking water to millions of refugees around the world. http://www.earth-water.org/.

Thirsty Planet, United Kingdom: A brand of bottled water that raises money for the provision of clean water in Africa. A portion of the profit from each bottle is given to the charity Pump Aid. http://www.thirsty-planet.com/.

Athena Bottled Water, United States: This small bottler produces bottled water in order to raise funds to battle breast cancer. One hundred percent of the net profits from the purchase of Athena water are devoted to finding a cure. http://www.athenapartners.org/.

Nika Bottled Water, United States: Nika directs 100 percent of its profits to help meet water and sanitation needs in impoverished countries. The company derives its name from a Zulu word meaning "to give." http://www.nikawater.org/.

from that, Goose traveled around the world and saw firsthand the challenges of poverty and the role that safe and clean water play in improving people's quality of life. On returning to England, Goose created One Water, which now has production lines in Britain, Ireland, South Africa, Malaysia, Australia, and the United States. In 2007 the company reported that profits of over £260,000 were used to build water pumps in African communities; by late 2008 over £1.4 million had been raised. In May 2007 Goose was named a "Great Briton" and was recognized for his work by the Queen in a ceremony alongside Helen Mirren, Geri Halliwell, and David Beckham.[7] In November 2008 Goose was named Credit Suisse Entrepreneur of the Year at the National Business Awards.[8]

The campaign against bottled water has added some unusual commercial twists too. In 2005, an organization in the Netherlands began offering Neau (pronounced "no" in Dutch) water bottles in a public campaign against commercial mineral waters. "Take Neau for an answer," the campaign ads proclaimed, and "Neau thirst." The bottle is designed to be refilled at taps, while profits from the sales of Neau water bottles are sent to water projects in developing countries.9

Critics may chafe at the apparent contradiction of selling bottled water under an ethical moniker. Some see efforts to market "green" bottled water as simply greenwashing—an attempt to do ethically or environmentally what shouldn't be done at all. Fiji Water's efforts to position themselves as the most environmentally responsible bottled water prompted the American Public Media's Greenwash Brigade to award them a top 2008 Greenwash prize, noting the massive energy cost required to transport Fiji water to market, the evils of producing and disposing of plastics, and problems with the company's claim of "carbon neutrality."10

Some groups argue for banning bottled water or restricting sales in certain markets, or even eliminating bottled water completely.11 If the complete elimination of bottled water were desirable and achievable, such an ideologically pure position might be supportable. But in the meantime, I think that even a modest expansion of hitherto inadequate efforts to help meet basic human needs for water, supported by the intentional or unintentional contributions of millions of bottled water consumers, has some merit, if efforts to produce an "ethical" bottled water are not simply greenwashing. Indeed, if each of the over 30 billion liters of bottled water sold in the United States in 2008 contributed the same 5 cents to water projects in needy regions that Ethos Water contributes, over $1.5 billion would have been raised. This would be a huge amount of money for safe water projects—far more than the entire annual U.S. foreign aid budget for water and sanitation worldwide. Spent effectively, this money could go a long way toward preventing bottled water use in developing countries by providing a safe, cheap, equitable alternative for the world's poorest people. If bottled water isn't going to disappear, then maybe the biggest problem with ethical bottled water is that there isn't more of it.

CHAPTER 12

The Future of Water

Making predictions is very difficult, especially about the future.
— Casey Stengel, famous philosopher (and Major
League Baseball legend)

It is one thing to find fault with an existing system. It is another thing
altogether, a more difficult task, to replace it with another approach
that is better.
— Nelson Mandela, speaking of water resource
management[I]

THE WORLD'S rapidly growing dependence on expensive, commercial bottled water is a symptom of the fundamental failure to provide safe and affordable drinking water to everyone on the planet—which should be a basic human right. Those of us who live in the richer nations of the world are buying more and more bottled water because we increasingly fear or dislike our tap water, we distrust governments to regulate, monitor, and protect public water systems adequately, we can't find public fountains anywhere anymore, we are convinced by advertisers and marketers that bottled water will make us healthier, thinner, or stronger, and we're told that it is just another benign consumer "choice." If we let our tap water systems decay, however, soon bottled water won't be a choice—it will be a necessity, as it is already is in countries without safe tap water.

At the same time, the growing revolution against bottled water is public recognition that safe and affordable water for all, under public control and protection, is a goal worth fighting for. Our relationship to water must change; indeed, it is changing already. We are in the midst of a critical transition and the path we choose in the next few years will determine whether we move toward a world of safe, expensive water for the privileged and wealthy in the form of bottled water or private water systems, or toward more comprehensive safe water for all.

This is not the first such transition. Humanity's approach to dealing with fresh water has evolved over the eons, through two distinct Ages of Water. I believe we are in the midst of a transition to a third approach, one that is fundamentally new. The First Water Age began when *Homo sapiens* emerged from the mists of evolution as thinking beings and began the transition from primitive hunter/gatherer societies. During this age, water was simply taken when needed and available. The natural hydrologic cycle of evaporation, condensation, precipitation, and runoff all worked to purify water, and the rivers, streams, lakes, and springs fed by rain were usually safe to drink. If the water was too dirty, early humans got sick and died. But life, as Thomas Hobbes observed, was already nasty, brutish, and short.

The Second Water Age began when humans started to organize into more formal fixed communities and to outgrow the limits of local water resources. During this age, we see the first intentional manipulation of the hydrologic cycle. And we see it everywhere in the archeological record, especially in arid, desert regions. It is no accident that many of the greatest early civilizations arose on the banks of perennial rivers, like the Tigris, Euphrates, Indus, Ganges, Yangtze, Yellow, Colorado, Nile, and Jordan. Where there was water, there was life. And where there were growing communities, there was the need to develop water-management systems and institutions. Ancient civilizations left behind traces of irrigation canals, early dams to store or divert water, aqueducts and *acequias* that move water tens and even hundreds of kilometers with only the force of gravity, and the earliest wastewater systems to separate good water from bad. These early cultures also gave us the first laws and social structures for managing water. The Code of Hammurabi, written by the great early king of ancient Babylon over 3,000 years ago, lays out some of the first laws and rules governing the rational and fair management of precious irrigation water and the maintenance of water systems, including punishments for water theft.

The Second Water Age reached full flower in the nineteenth and twentieth centuries when societies began to master the natural hydrologic cycle in order to provide clean water and to recycle our wastes using chemical, mechanical, biological, and institutional tools that mimic and amplify nature's power. The Second Water Age is characterized by massive physical interventions in the natural hydrologic cycle. We built huge dams to capture water in wet periods to use in dry periods, and systems of canals and aqueducts to move water thousands of kilometers from wet regions to dry regions. Our cities rely on complex systems of pumps, treatment plants, distribution pipelines, wastewater collection systems, and waste-treatment plants. If these systems were to fail, our cities would fail as well.

All of our engineered water-treatment processes that flocculate, coagulate, precipitate, condense, and distill water are mechanical imitations of natural processes. We build massive sand or charcoal or mechanical filters that mimic the purification role played by soils. We run water through reverse-osmosis membranes that imitate the way cell walls separate salts from solution. We pass water under high-intensity ultraviolet lamps that replicate the purifying effects of the sun. We grow vats of naturally occurring waste-eating bacteria that take the biological products we excrete and consume them, producing fertilizer, oxygen, and energy. We use fossil fuels to distill water in massive boilers and condensers that are concentrated mechanical reproductions of the hydrologic cycle. And all of these artificial interventions are necessary because the population of the planet has outgrown the ability of nature to provide adequate water for our needs and to purify our wastes.

We are now, I believe, at the beginning of another transition, this time to the Third Water Age. The Second Age brought enormous benefits to us, but has ultimately proven inadequate to the growing need. Billions of people still suffer unnecessary water-related diseases because they lack safe water and sanitation. Aquatic ecosystems are dying due to our use, diversion, and contamination of the fresh water they too need to survive. The risks of political, economic, and military conflicts over water resources are growing. Climate change is already starting to alter basic hydrological conditions around the world. And the technological "hard path" fixes we applied in the Second Water Age seem less and less likely to solve these problems by themselves. The growing use of bottled water is evidence that the old ways of managing water challenges are putting us on the wrong side of history.

We must do more than just "more of the same" if we are going to truly address global water problems. We must make the transition to the Third Water Age by following a more sustainable approach that recognizes the realities of a renewable but ultimately limited resource. This approach is what I have called the "soft path for water."[2] The soft path for water is a comprehensive approach to sustainable water use and management that takes advantage of the remarkable engineering skills and technologies available for managing water but also looks to tools like the proper application of economics, innovative incentives for efficient water use, appropriate regulatory approaches for protecting water quality and ecosystem health, and expanded public participation in decision-making.

A key objective of the soft path is to meet the water-related *needs* of people and businesses, rather than merely supplying water. The use of water must be considered a means to an end, not an end in and of itself. People want to be clean or to clean their clothes or produce food and other goods and services using convenient, cost-effective, and socially acceptable means. They don't have an ideological preference, or shouldn't, for how much water is used, and in many cases may not care whether water is used at all. If there are ways to reduce the demand for water while continuing to provide these goods and services, overall pressures on the world's water supply will fall.

The soft path also requires that we match the quality of water needed with the quality that is available. Higher-quality water should be reserved for those uses that *require* higher quality. The soft path recognizes that ecological health and the activities that depend on it (e.g., fishing, swimming, tourism, delivery of clean raw water to downstream users) are fundamental, not peripheral, to water management. The soft path recognizes the complexity of water economics, including the power of economies of scale and scope and recognizes that investments in small-scale, decentralized solutions can be just as cost-effective as investments in large, centralized options. Finally, the soft path requires water providers to interact closely with water users and to effectively engage community groups in water management. These ideas contrast and conflict with the fundamental assumptions of the Second Water Age that water left in a river or lake or aquifer is not being used productively, and that large-scale central water infrastructure is the only realistic way to meet demands.

Bottled water is a consequence of the failure of the "hard path," and the growing backlash against it is a symptom of the need for a new paradigm. If everyone on the planet had access to affordable safe tap water, bottled water use would be seen as unnecessary. If government regulatory agencies actually worked to protect the public from poor-quality water, false advertising, misleading marketing, and blatant hucksterism, sales of magic water elixirs would be halted. If public sources of drinking water were more accessible, arguments about the convenience of bottled water would seem silly. And if bottled water companies had to incorporate the true economic and environmental costs of the production and disposal of plastic bottles, as well as the extraction and use of sensitive groundwater, into the price of their product, sales would plummet.

Machiavellian motives can be inferred from the dramatic expansion of bottled water in the last decade: Some claim that it is an orchestrated effort to privatize precious water resources and to turn water from a natural right into a luxury, a commercial product. Certainly, the bottled water industry is successfully capitalizing on, and profiting from, the decay of our comprehensive safe drinking water systems, or, in the poorer countries of the world, their complete absence. But motives aside, society must not abandon municipal systems, or let the rich fall back on individual point-of-use systems that purify water just for those who can afford it, or try to provide everyone with bottled water for their potable water needs. The answer is to continue to build new and innovative water and wastewater systems, expand and maintain the remarkable water systems we've already built, get the failing pipes and lead contamination out of old · buildings, and learn to manage water for the long-term future, not the next quarterly earnings period.

Pursuing these goals won't eliminate the bottled water industry. Consumers will always seek a diversity of choices, including the choice to buy water in convenient, single-serve containers. But the bottled water industry itself is in need of serious reform and comprehensive regulation in order to safeguard human health, reduce the environmental impacts of bottling and transporting water, and protect the public from misrepresentations and lies about unproven health benefits of bottled water.

Let me offer two simple but diametrically opposed visions of the future.

In the first vision, the poorest parts of the world never get the high-quality reliable water systems developed in Europe and the United States, and even these water systems are allowed to decay to the point where no one trusts the quality of tap water for drinking. In this vision, the quality of the water from our faucets deteriorates, and safe drinking water is increasingly available only in fancy and expensive bottled water and individual point-of-use systems for the rich. Water is privatized, commoditized, and controlled for those who can afford it, and bottled water sales expand everywhere, for the demand is high. Billions of poor are left to rely on drinking water from private vendors, poorly run and regulated municipal systems, dubious tap water, water bottlers, or contaminated local sources. Cholera, dysentery, and typhoid resurge in the slums and under-served cities of the world. Scarcity and contamination continue to expand, ecosystems lose more and more of the water they need to survive, and inequities and conflicts over water worsen. No doubt many readers already recognize all this as a vision of much of the world as it already is for billions. And it is a vision of where the United States is heading if the philosophies of anti-tax, anti-government, and anti-regulation are allowed to continue to cripple municipal infrastructure of all kinds and weaken government enforcement of water-quality protections. The front-page news in September 2009 that drinking water standards in many parts of the United States have not been adequately monitored or enforced was only news to those who haven't been paying attention.

But there is good news as well, enough to suggest an alternative vision of the future. In this second vision, the world moves toward sustainably managed freshwater resources, where every person on the planet has safe and reliable drinking water, ecosystems and communities all have their basic water needs satisfied, and water is used efficiently and carefully. Water-related diseases, conquered in the richer nations a hundred years ago, are conquered for all. Water quality is protected and water-quality laws are strengthened and enforced for all. Aquatic ecosystems around the world are restored and once again provide natural water purification services. And conflicts over water are resolved with negotiation, discussion, and public debate. In this second vision, bottled water doesn't disappear, but it once again becomes what it used to be—a luxury bought and consumed only for reasons of pretention, style, and occasional convenience, or as a short-term solution for emergencies when other safe alternatives are not available.

I believe this second vision is inevitable—that we will sooner or later have no choice but to solve our water problems. We're already moving toward the soft path, but we have a long way to go, and we may take many missteps along the way. If we're to have a chance of making the journey successfully, five serious reforms of the water industry are needed:

- *Support and expand state-of-the-art tap water systems.* Towns and cities must continue to invest in building and operating the best municipal tap water systems that technology and money can produce. Bottled water, like any product, can only thrive when there isn't a better alternative. We must make sure there always is. The technology exists to provide inexpensive water of the highest purity. We can still pursue a future where all municipal water systems operate the best water-purification systems available with consistent, independent, and reliable water-quality testing. Old distribution systems, which often add contaminants or poor taste to tap water, must be upgraded and replaced, including all old plumbing connections that leach lead or other contaminants into otherwise safe water. Public water fountains can be restored, and modern "hydration stations" with modern filters and regular maintenance can be installed widely, to provide safe and free water in our schools, parks, and other public spaces.

- *Develop, pass, and enforce smarter water regulations.* New water-quality regulations must be enacted and vigorously enforced to close the massive loopholes that permit bottlers to meet different standards than those in place for tap water. In the United States, there should be a complete overhaul of the Food and Drug Administration, which seems uninterested, unwilling, or unable to adequately enforce and monitor bottled water quality. If this is not possible, the responsibility for regulating bottled water must be taken away from the FDA and given to an agency that will do the job. No matter which agency is responsible, the same water-quality standards and testing and reporting requirements should be applied to both bottled water and tap water. All water-quality standards must be upgraded, testing rules for both bottled water and tap water must be tightened, tests must be done by completely independent laboratories, and all results must be promptly and publicly reported.

• *Require truthful labeling.* Labeling of all bottled water must identify the source of the water, the mineral content, the processes used to purify the water, the name, location, and phone number of the bottler, and information on where up-to-date water-quality test results can be found. This same information must also be posted on websites for each water bottler. The current FDA nutrition label, which hides far more than it reveals, should not be used for bottled water. Regulations to require truth in branding and labeling should be strengthened and enforced.

• *Protect consumers from fraud and misrepresentations.* Government agencies responsible for protecting consumers against fraudulent and misleading advertising and marketing must actually work to protect consumers. In the United States, this means that the FTC and the FDA must aggressively move against the twenty-first-century snake-oil salesmen and medicine-show hucksters who are misleading the public about the potential of some bottled waters to cure their medical ills, help them lose weight, or otherwise magically solve their problems. This will require far more serious efforts to crack down on advertising fraud, especially on the Internet.

• *Reduce bottled water's environmental impact.* The environmental consequences of producing and using bottled water can be minimized by reducing the energy costs associated with making and transporting bottled water and by aggressively dealing with plastic waste. I urge people to adopt a "drink local" philosophy to match the growing movement to "eat local." Drinking imported bottled water is especially costly to consumers and the environment because of the massive energy costs of moving water from one place to another. Bottlers must be required to substantially boost the recycled plastic content of their bottles. The industry must stop describing plastic bottles as "recyclable" as though that were

the end of their responsibility, and they should support comprehensive efforts to actually recycle plastic bottles. All of them. Recycling programs should be expanded with the target of capturing
and reusing 100 percent of PET and other recyclable plastics.

In the end, the debate about bottled water is really a debate
about the value of water, human rights versus responsibilities, environmental priorities and protection, economic markets versus public
goods, government intervention versus government reform, and
more. If we are thoughtful, however, we will see bottled water for
what it is—the result of a failure to provide satisfactory public water
systems and services for everyone—and realize that our obsession
with bottled water can be overcome if we address the reasons people
seek it out.

Now I think I'll go get a glass of tap water.

Acknowledgments

MANY PEOPLE played a part in the creation of this book. Friends, colleagues, and industry representatives generously shared data and information with me. Researchers and reporters dug up stories about bottled water use, or companies, or controversies. A few government officials and company employees were willing to send me reports or numbers that are not typically available to the public. Community activists offered their stories and experiences with local bottled water controversies and actions. Other scientists reviewed my descriptions of hydrologic processes and my analysis of trends. And—day after day—my family members put up with the stories I told, the complaints I uttered, and the excuses I made for another late dinner or another trip out of town. It is hard to thank them all, but I will try to do so now, even if I inadvertently leave some names out.

First and foremost (rather than last but not least), I couldn't have done this without my wife Nicki Norman, who serves as sounding board and a voice of rationality and moderation, and who sees the big picture when I'm up to my eyeballs in details. What can I say other than thank you, thank you, thank you. And the same to my sons Daniel and Jeremy, who put up with my ramblings and musings, and who, with their sharp insights, often cleared up a foggy idea of mine.

Special thanks to Pamela Matson and her husband Peter Vitousek, who generously offered their secluded rainforest hideaway where, over the course of several weeks, many of the ideas, stories, and angles of the book took shape. And thanks to their closest neighbors, whose wireless signal I poached.

Thanks to my agent, Kimberly Witherspoon of Inkwell, and especially to my longtime Island Press editor Todd Baldwin for his support, direction, and thoughtful, clarifying edits. Michael Fleming also offered many thoughtful comments and clarifying edits.

Many other people offered data and ideas on the complex nature of the bottled water industry. Not everyone on this list will like what I've written; indeed, some may be outraged, but I thank them nevertheless for talking with me, sharing information, and expressing their views. This book reflects my opinions, of course, not theirs.

Ron Baird, Maude Barlow, Jeff Belchamber, Marty Bourque, Jody Clarke, Heather Cooley, Vanessa D'Cruz, Nick Dege, Joe Doss, Pat Franklin, Brian Germann, Robert Glennon, Jonathan Greenblatt, Gerald Haraguchi, Matt Heberger, Gary Hemphill, Wayne Houseright, Brian Howard, Yutaka Ishiyama, Bruce Karas, Susan Kattchee, Leonard F. Konikow, Kyle Kunst, David Langer, Janet Larsen, Larry Lawrence, Tania Levy, Kully Lindstrom, Angela Logomasini, Steve Lower, Zoe Maggio, Lisa Manley, Janet McDonald, Alex McIntosh, Patty Moore, Benjamin Morse, Jim Olson, Keith Olson, Pranav Padhiar, Heidi Paul, Will Peakin, Daniel Pellegrom, Alex Prud'homme, Fred Ramberg, Kristen Reinhardt, David Richardson, Maggie Rodgers, Nancy Ross, Elizabeth Royte, Andrew Schneider, Jeff Seabright, Courtney Smith, Doug Spitzer, Richard Stevens, Mel Suffet, Harvey Tanaka, Peter Thum, Dan Vermeer, David Weiman, Dora Wong.

Notes

Endnotes, Chapter 1

1. See UCF press release of July 11, 2005, by Tom Evelyn (http://www.wesh .com/news/14143574/detail.html?rss=orl&psp=news), stating that the Board "has not yet formally voted on whether to build the stadium." Similarly, in a March 31, 2005, presentation to the UCF Board of Trustees by the stadium architects 360 Architecture, all permitting for the stadium was to be complete no earlier than July 2005, well after implementation of the 2004 building codes. "Code group: University of Central Florida didn't adhere to drinking water rules," *Orlando Sentinel*, September 22, 2007 (from http://www.water webster.com/BottledWater.htm, accessed August 10, 2008). See also Table 403.1 of the 2004 Florida Building Code, which states that stadiums (A-5 category buildings) must have one water fountain per 1000 occupants. The requirement seems to be the same in the 2001 Florida Plumbing Code, Table 403.1, chap. 4, p.4.1 (see http://www2.iccsafe.org/states/Florida2001/FL _Plumbing/FL_Plumbing.htm).
2. UCF To Install Water Fountains in New Stadium (video), http://www.youtube .com/watch?v=4t-44S_gebI&feature=related (accessed September 18, 2007).
3. Luis Zaragoza and Claudia Zequeira, "UCF in hot water with fans: Stadium has no drinking fountains; students thirsty for answers," *Orlando Sentinel*, September 18, 2007.
4. See http://drinkingfountains.org/.
5. See http://borregospringsbottledwater.com/waterfaq.php (accessed September 12, 2008).
6. Dave Carpenter, "Thirsty for utter dominance, Gatorade declares war on tap water," *Denver Post*, May 28, 2000.
7. See http://www.time.com/time/magazine/article/0,9171,91374,00.html (accessed September 19, 2008).
8. Brendan Buhler, "Convention Crashing: The International Bottled Water Association," *Las Vegas Sun*, October 9, 2006.
9. *Brandweek*, "Aquafina Employs Kudrow to Tout 'Nothing' Campaign," July 2, 2001, http://findarticles.com/p/articles/mi_moBDW/is_27_42/ai_76443142 (accessed December 10, 2009).
10. International Bottled Water Association New Release, "ABC News 20/20 is Wrong About Bottled Water," May 7, 2005.
11. Quoted in Jonathan Fowler, "Study: Bottled Water Not Better," Associated Press, May 2, 2001.
12. See http://www.fda.gov/FDAC/features/2002/402_h2o.html (accessed September 12, 2008).

13. Australasian Bottled Water Association website, http://www.bottledwater.org
.au/scripts/cgiip.exe/WService=ASP0003/ccms.r?PageId=5002 (accessed December 10, 2009).

14. On its website (www.cei.org/about) the CEI describes itself as "a public interest group dedicated to free enterprise and limited government," accessed December 10, 2009.

15. Fred Smith, e-mail to author, October 21, 2007.

16. See http://enjoybottledwater.org/?p=85 (accessed September 15, 2009).

17. Jody Clarke (CEI), e-mail to author, September 17, 2008.

18. The Coca-Cola Company, "The Olive Gardens targets tap water, and wins!" from http://cockeyed.com/coke/html/olivegard_article_ss2.html (downloaded August 21, 2001). See also David Gallagher, "Having customers say no to tap water," *New York Times*, August 21, 2001.

19. See http://www.stayfreemagazine.org/public/coke_story.html (accessed September 10, 2008). Quotation from metafilter.com, http://www.metafilter.com/9399/ (accessed December 10, 2009).

20. See http://findarticles.com/p/articles/mi_m0BQE/is_4_17/ai_n16374556/print (accessed September 10, 2008).

21. See, for example, Brita's full-page ad in *New York* magazine on January 16, 1995, entitled "We'd like to clear up a few things about tap water" (22), or the Brita ad in the October 2003 issue of *Ebony* magazine describing their water pitcher that "turns tap water into drinking water" (146).

22. "Canadian Advertising Success Stories 2007: Brita," http://www.cassies.ca/winners/2007Winners/winners_brita.html (accessed December 10, 2009).

23. Advertising Standards Canada, "Ad Complaint Reports—Q3 2006," http://www.adstandards.com/en/Standards/adComplaintsReports.asp?periodquarter=3&periodyear=2006 (accessed December 10, 2009).

24. Brian Howard, "Despite the hype, bottled water is neither cleaner nor greener than tap water," *E—The Environmental Magazine*, December 9, 2003, http://www.commondreams.org/headlines03/1209-10.htm (accessed December 10, 2009).

25. Gregory Karp, "The Morning Call: Tap water might fit your bill better than bottled," *Chicago Tribune*, September 10, 2006. Also, see Kay's quote at http://a.abcnews.com/WNT/Story?id=131639&page=2 (accessed March 16, 2009).

26. Written Testimony of Joseph K. Doss, President and CEO, International Bottled Water Association Before the Domestic Policy Subcommittee of the Oversight and Government Reform Committee of the United States House of Representatives. Hearing on "Assessing the Environmental Risks of the Water Bottling Industry's Extraction of Groundwater," Washington, D.C., December 12, 2007.

Endnotes, Chapter 2

1. Burn On. Words and music by RANDY NEWMAN © 1970 (renewed) UNICHAPPELL MUSIC INC. All rights reserved. Used by permission of ALFRED PUBLISHING CO., INC.

2. *CNNMoney.com*, "Crisp. Refreshing. And only ever-so-slightly poisonous . . . ,"

http://money.cnn.com/galleries/2007/biz2/0701/gallery.101dumbest_2007/20
.html (accessed December 11, 2009).

3. See http://penelope.uchicago.edu/Thayer/E/Roman/Texts/secondary/
   SMIGRA*/Aquaeductus.html.
4. Stephanie Pope, "The Muse, Part 2: The Fountain of Youth," http://www.myth
   opoetry.com/mythopoetics/essay_muse_two.html (accessed December 11, 2009).
5. Charles Dickens Jr., "Drinking Fountains," *Dickens's Dictionary of London*
   (London: Charles Dickens and Evans, 1879).
6. Detroit Water and Sewage Department, "The First 300 Years," http://www
   .dwsd.org/history/complete_history.pdf (accessed May 25, 2009).
7. *New York Times*, "P. T. Barnum's gift to Bethel," August 26, 1881.
8. "Bradford's and Winslow's Journal," originally printed in London, 1622.
   Reprinted in *A Library of American Literature*, vol. 1, compiled and edited by
   E. C. Stedman and E. M. Hutchinson (New York: Charles L. Webster and
   Company, 1889).
9. John Burnett, *Liquid Pleasures: A Social History of Drinks in Modern Britain* (London: Routledge, 1999).
10. Bruce Haley, *The Healthy Body and Victorian Culture* (Cambridge, MA: Harvard
    University Press, 1978).
11. Charles E. Rosenberg, *The Cholera Years: The United States in 1832, 1849, and
    1866* (Chicago: University of Chicago Press, 1987).
12. David Cutler and Grant Miller, "The Role of Public Health Improvements
    in Health Advances: The Twentieth-Century United States," *Demography* 42,
    no. 1 (February 2005): 1–22.
13. The Act does not apply to private wells serving fewer than 25 people. EPA estimates that these wells serve around 10 percent of the U.S. population. Some
    states set standards for these wells directly.
14. *The Daily Mail* (London), "Revealed: 250,000 people left without clean drinking water after a rabbit infected supply," July 15, 2008, http://www.mailon
    sunday.co.uk/news/article-1035252/Revealed-250-000-people-left-clean
    -drinking-water-RABBIT-infected-supply.html (accessed December 11, 2009).

Endnotes, Chapter 3

1. IBWA website, updated May 27, 2004, http://www.bottledwater.org/public/
   BWFactsHome_main.htm (accessed August 2008).
2. Corporate Accountability International, "Think Outside the Bottle" Campaign, http://www.stopcorporateabuse.org/cms/page1544.cfm (accessed May 2,
   2009).
3. Massachusetts Legislature, "An Act against selling unwholesome Provisions,"
   passed March 8, 1785. (Illustration from John P. Swann, "FDA's Origin,"
   http://www.fda.gov/AboutFDA/WhatWeDo/History/Origin/ucm124403.htm
   [accessed December 11, 2009].)
4. United States Code of Federal Regulations, 21 CFR Part 110.
5. Public Health Security and Bioterrorism Preparedness and Response (Bioterrorism) Act of 2002, Pub. L. No. 107–188, 116 Stat. 605 (2002).
6. Federal Food, Drug, and Cosmetic Act § 410, 21 U.S.C. § 349 (2005).

7. Speech to the Beverage Forum in New York, May 21, 2008, http://www
.beveagemarketing.com/BeverageForum2008_KimJeffery.html (accessed
October 2008).
8. Corporate Accountability International website, http://www.stopcorporate
abuse.org/content/bottled-water-industry-threatening-human-right-water
(accessed March 15, 2009).
9. See http://recipes.howstuffworks.com/bottled-water.htm/printable (accessed
October 20, 2008).
10. Environmental Protection Agency, 1989 Total Coliform Rule, http://www
.epa.gov/ogwdw000/disinfection/tcr/regulation.html (accessed December 11,
2009). See also: "Total Coliform Rule Overview: Total Coliform Rule/
Distribution System Rule Webcast," January 17, 2007, http://www.epa.gov/
ogwdw000/disinfection/tcr/pdfs/trainingmaterials/training_tcr_01172007_tcro
verview.pdf (accessed December 11, 2009).
11. Federal Register, May 29, 2009, http://edocket.access.gpo.gov/2009/E912494
.htm (accessed May 29, 2009).
12. Department of Health and Human Services, FDA Proposed Rules Docket No.
FDA-2008-N-0446 for 21 CFR Parts 129 and 165, http://edocket.access.gpo
.gov/2008/pdf/E8-21619.pdf.
13. Coliform at EU standards:
    1.3. Criteria for microbiological analyses at source. These analyses must include—
    1.3.1. demonstration of the absence of parasites and pathogenic microorganisms;
    1.3.2. quantitative determination of the revivable colony count indicative of faecal
        contamination—
        (a) the absence of *Escherichia coli* and other coliforms in 250 millilitres at 37°C
            and 44.5°C;
        (b) the absence of faecal streptococci in 250 millilitre.
            (From the EU website, http://eur-lex.europa.eu/LexUriServ/LexUriServ.do
            ?uri=OJ:L:2009:164:0045:0058:EN:PDF [accessed December 11, 2009].)
14. Quotation from testimony by Joshua M. Sharfstein, Principal Deputy Commissioner and Acting Commissioner, Food and Drug Administration (FDA)
before the Committee on Energy and Commerce, Subcommittee on Oversight
and Investigations, United States House of Representatives, July 08, 2009,
http://www.hhs.gov/asl/testify/2009/07/t20090708a.html (accessed December 12, 2009).
15. See FDA Regulations on Quality Compliance, 21CFR129.80 (g)(1), Section
165.110(b). Also, see Lauren Posnick and Henry Kim, "Bottled Water Regulation and the FDA," in *Food and Safety Magazine*, August/September 2002,
reproduced in http://www.fda.gov/downloads/Food/FoodSafety/Product
-Specific-Information/BottledWaterCarbonatedSoftDrinks/ucm077094
.pdf (accessed December 12, 2009).
16. Michigan's Drinking Water, http://www.gem.msu.edu/gw/btl_wtr.html (accessed
October 20, 2008).
17. United States Code of Federal Regulations, 21 CFR 129.35.
18. United States Code of Federal Regulations, 21 CFR 129.3.
19. United States Code of Federal Regulations, 21 CFR 165.110(c).

20. U.S. Government Accountability Office, "U.S. Needs a Single Agency to Administer a Unified, Risk-Based Inspection System," GAO/T-RCED-99-256 (Washington, DC: U.S. Government Printing Office, 1999).

21. U.S. Government Accountability Office, "Bottled Water: FDA Safety and Consumer Protections Are Often Less Stringent Than Comparable EPA Protections for Tap Water," GAO-09-610 (Washington, DC: U.S. Government Printing Office, June 2009).

22. "Lawmakers pledge to move on FDA reform in the next Congress," http:// pharmtech.findpharma.com/pharmtech/Manufacturing/Lawmakers-Pledge-to -Move-on-FDA-Reform-in-the-ext/ArticleStandard/Article/detail/569452 ?contextCategoryId=35097 (accessed December 4, 2008).

23. President Barack Obama, Weekly Address, March 14, 2009, http://www .whitehouse.gov/blog/09/03/14/Food-Safety (accessed December 11, 2009).

24. U.S. Food and Drug Administration, Center for Food Safety and Applied Nutrition, "FDA Recall Policies," Industry Affairs Staff Brochure, June 2002, http://vm.cfsan.fda.gov/~lrd/recall2.html (accessed May 1, 2008).

25. A comprehensive summary, with dates, names, locations, and types of contamination, is now posted on the website of the Pacific Institute (www.pacinst.org).

26. Quoted in Michael D. White, *A Short Course in International Marketing Blunders* (Novato, CA: World Trade Press, 2002), 18.

27. Ibid., 21.

28. George James, "Perrier Recalls Its Water in U.S. After Benzene Is Found in Bottles," *New York Times*, February 10, 1990, http://query.nytimes.com/gst/ fullpage.html?sec=health&res=9C0CE7D61F39F933A25751C0A966958260 (accessed December 11, 2009).

29. RTE News, "E. coli found in Bottled water: FSA," November 17, 2008, http:// www.rte.ie/news/2008/1117/water.html (accessed November 30, 2008). See also Shane Phelan, "Bottled water scare as dangerous germs found," *Irish Independent*, November 17, 2007, http://www.independent.ie/national-news/bottled -water-scare-as-dangerous-germs-found-1541957.html (accessed November 30, 2008).

30. Shane Phelan, "Watchdog lashed in water row," *Irish Independent*, December 5, 2008, http://www.independent.ie/national-news/watchdog-lashed-in-water -row1564572.html (accessed December 24, 2008).

31. Megan Rauscher, "'High Levels' of Bacteria Found in Bottled Water," Reuters, March 11, 2004, http://www.purebev.com/in_the_news.php (accessed December 12, 2009).

32. *Daily Times* (of Pakistan), March 9, 2003, http://www.dailytimes.com.pk/ default.asp?page=story_9-3-2003_pg5_2 (accessed December 12, 2009).

33. Rajeev Syal, "Test targets cheats who sell tap water by the bottle," *Times* (London), January 20, 2007, http://www.timesonline.co.uk/tol/news/uk/ article1294654.ece (accessed December 12, 2009).

34. *Thanh Nien News*, "Paraffin in water poisoned school children," May 16, 2006, http://www.thanhniennews.com/healthy/?catid=8&newsid=15510 (accessed December 12, 2009).

35. Raymund F. Antonio. "Manila warns on bottled water," *Manila Bulletin*

Online, October 7, 2006, http://www.mb.com.ph/node/95895 (accessed December 12, 2009).

Endnotes, Chapter 4

1. Brian Clark Howard, "Message in a Bottle: Despite the Hype, Bottled Water Is Neither Cleaner nor Greener Than Tap Water," E—*The Environmental Magazine*, September/October 2003, http://www.emagazine.com/view/?1125 (accessed July 22, 2008).
2. Sherri Day, "Suit Disputes Integrity of Poland Spring Water," *New York Times*, June 20, 2003, http://www.nytimes.com/2003/06/20/business/suit-disputes -integrity-of-poland-spring-water.html (accessed September 9, 2009).
3. Ibid.
4. Anthony Brooks, "Poland Spring Settles Class-Action Lawsuit," National Public Radio, September 3, 2003, http://www.npr.org/templates/story/story.php ?storyId=1419713 (accessed November 12, 2009).
5. United States Code of Federal Regulations, 21 CFR § 165.110 (a).
6. United States Code, 21 USC § 343(g)(1).
7. Directive 96/70/EC of the European Parliament relating to the exploitation and marketing of natural mineral waters, 1996 and amendments, http://eurlex .europa.eu/LexUriServ/LexUriServ.do?uri=CELEX:31996L0070:EN:HTML (accessed December 12, 2009). Part 3, 11(2) requires "spring" waters to satisfy all labeling requirements of Part 2, Section 8(3) for mineral waters.
8. Jason Blevins, "Nestle plan sets off water war," *The Denver Post*, March 23, 2009, http://www.denverpost.com/ news/ci_11974140 (accessed December 12, 2009).
9. Vinnee Tong, "Aquafina Labels: It's Tap Water," Associated Press, July 27, 2007; see, for example, http://www.theglobeandmail.com/news/world/article772319 .ece (accessed December 12, 2009).
10. Brian Clark Howard, "Message in a Bottle: Despite the Hype, Bottled Water Is Neither Cleaner nor Greener Than Tap Water," E—*The Environmental Magazine*, September/October 2003, http://www.emagazine.com/view/?1125 (accessed July 22, 2008).
11. "Understanding Dasani," www.dasani.com (accessed before June 2003); see also http://web.archive.org/web/20010124012800/http://dasani.com/.
12. U.S. Government Accountability Office, "Bottled Water: FDA Safety and Consumer Protections Are Often Less Stringent Than Comparable EPA Protections for Tap Water," GAO-09-610 (Washington, DC: U.S. Government Printing Office, June 2009).
13. "Vended Water," California Senate Bill S220, http://info.sen.ca.gov/pub/ 07-08/bill/sen/sb_0201-0250/sb_220_bill_20071013_chaptered.pdf (accessed December 11, 2009).
14. "Around the Water Cooler: California follow-up: SB 220 and labeling," *Water Technology Magazine* 30, no. 6 (June 2007), http://www.waternet.com/article .asp?IndexID=6636763 (accessed December 9, 2008).
15. According to former FDA official Fred Degnan, now on the bottlers' side: "There is no room on the label of a bottled water product for a complete and

clear explanation of the significance or insignificance to consumers' health of the presence of contaminants in the product." See Frank Greve, "American's thirst for bottled water growing from the tap, it's safe and costs pennies," Philadelphia Newspapers Inc., May 11, 1998, http://archives.foodsafety .ksu.edu/fsnet/ 1998/5-1998/fs-05-12-98-01.txt (accessed September 22, 2009). See also National Soft Drink Association, Comments on FDA Docket No. 97N-0436 ("given the limited amount of available label space . . ."), April 24, 2000, http://www.fda.gov/ohrms/dockets/dailys/00/apr00/042600/ c000064.pdf (accessed December 12, 2009).

16. Natalie Zmuda, "Why Bottled Water Is Not All Washed Up," *Advertising Age*, December 8, 2008, http://adage.com/cmostrategy/article?article_id=132992 (accessed February 19, 2008).

Endnotes, Chapter 5

1. Robert Glennon, *Water Follies* (Washington DC: Island Press, 2002), 30.

2. K. N. Eshleman, "Bottled Water Production in the United States: How Much Ground Water Is Actually Being Used?" Study Summary, Drinking Water Research Foundation, August 2004, http://www.dwrf.info/documents/ DWRFStudySummary-BWProductionandGroundwaterWithdrawalsv5 _000.doc (accessed September 9, 2006).

3. International Bottled Water Association, "IBWA Challenges Peter Gleick," 2005 Press Release, http://www.bottledwater.org/public/2004_Releases/ IBWA_Challenges_Peter_Gleick_Statements.html (accessed June 19, 2005).

4. Australasian Bottled Water Institute website, http://www.bottledwater.org.au/ scripts/cgiip.exe/WService=ASP0003/ccms.r?Roxy=0x0003176d&PageId =5002 (accessed May 25, 2009).

5. Letter from Absopure Corporation in opposition to Michigan Laws HB 4343 and HB 5065-73, December 2007, http://house.michigan.gov/SessionDocs/ 2007-2008/Testimony/Committee10-12-4-2007-2.pdf (accessed September 29, 2009).

6. New Hampshire Program of the American Friends Service Committee, Amicus Curiae Brief, N.H. Supreme Court No. 2004-0601, June 21, 2005, http://www .afsc.org/newhampshire/ht/a/GetDocumentAction/i/17849 (accessed December 12, 2009).

7. Thomas Ropp, "Firm told to stop tapping Seven Springs for bottled water," *Arizona Republic*, October 6, 2006; also "Water bottler feeling pressure: County demands business stop operation or face suit," *The Arizona Republic*, Oct. 7, 2006.

8. Michigan Citizens for Water Conservation v. Nestlé Waters North America, Inc., 709 N.W. 2d 174, pp. 194–98 (Mich. Ct. App. 2005), http://www .olemiss.edu/orgs/SGLC/National/SandBar/5.1bottled.htm (accessed December 12, 2009).

9. Department of Health and Human Services, FDA Proposed Rules Docket No. FDA-2008-N-0446 for 21 CFR Parts 129 and 165, http://edocket.access.gpo .gov/2008/pdf/E8-21619.pdf (accessed December 12, 2009).

10. *Federal Register*, May 29, 2009, http://edocket.access.gpo.gov/2009/E9 -12494.htm (accessed May 29, 2009).

11. Drinking Water Inspectorate, United Kingdom Department of the Environment, Transport, and Regions, "Cryptosporidium in Water Supplies," 2001, http://www.dwi.gov.uk/pubs/bouchier/bou004.htm (accessed January 2, 2009).

12. M. A. Di Benedetto, F. Di Piazza, C. M. Maida, A. Firenze, and R. Oliveri, "Occurrence of *Giardia* and *Cryptosporidium* in wastewater, surface water and ground water samples in Palermo (Sicily)" [Article in Italian], *Annali di igiene: medicina preventiva e di comunità* 17, no. 5 (September/October 2005):367–75, http://www.ncbi.nlm.nih.gov/sites/entrez?cmd=Retrieve&db=PubMed&list _uids=16353674&dopt=Abstract (accessed December 12, 2009).

13. R. de Carvalho Gamba, E. M. Prioli Ciapina, R. S. Espíndola, A. Pacheco, and V. H. Pellizari, "Detection of *Cryptosporidium sp.* Oocysts in Groundwater for Human Consumption in Itaquaquecetuba City, S. Paulo, Brazil," *Brazil Journal of Microbiology* 31, no. 2 (April/June 2000).

14. C. M. Hancock, J. B. Rose, and M. Callahan, "*Crypto* and *Giardia* in U.S. groundwater," *Journal of the American Water Works Association* 90, no. 3 (1998): 58–61.

15. C. Moulton-Hancock, J. B. Rose, G. J. Vasconcelos, S. I. Harris, P. T. Klonicki, and G. D. Sturbaum, "*Giardia* and *Cryptosporidium* occurrence in groundwater," *Journal of the American Water Works Association* 92, no. 9 (2000): 117–23.

Endnotes, Chapter 6

1. Brendan Buhler, "Convention Crashing: The International Bottled Water Association," *Las Vegas Sun*, October 9, 2006.

2. Chirag Trivedi, "People urged to ask for tap water," BBC News, February 19, 2008, http://news.bbc.co.uk/2/hi/uk_news/england/london/7252385.stm (accessed December 12, 2009).

3. Saxon East, October 9, 2006, www.yourlocalguardian.co.uk/misc/print.php ?artid=955599.

4. J. J. Moorman, *Mineral Springs of North America: How to Reach, and How to Use Them* (Philadelphia: J. B. Lippincott and Company, 1873).

5. J. K. Crook, *The Mineral Waters of the United States and Their Therapeutic Uses* (New York and Philadelphia: Lea Bros. & Co., 1899).

6. Juyun Lim and Harry T. Lawless, "Qualitative Differences of Divalent Salts: Multidimensional Scaling and Cluster Analysis," *Chemical Senses* 30, no. 9 (2005): 719–26.

7. Julie Arkell, "The World's First Water Sommelier," August 23, 2002, http://www.jancisrobinson.com/articles/jr846 (accessed December 12, 2009).

8. "Un cours d'eau pas comme les autres," http://www.labullebadoit.fr/ (accessed December 12, 2009).

9. Charles Bremner, "Paris Water Wars," *Times* (London), January 19, 2007, http://timescorrespondents.typepad.com/charles_bremner/2007/01/french_adv ertis.html#more (accessed December 12, 2009).

10. Tim Elliott, "A stiff drink. Virginality, minerality or gullibility? Why we spend $400 million a year on bottled water," *Sydney Morning Herald*, February 20, 2007, http://www.container-recycling.org/media/newsarticles/plastic/2007/ 2-20-Australia-AStiffDrink.htm (accessed December 12, 2009).

11. *Decanter.com*, Lucy Shaw, "Claridge's to sell water at £50 per litre," October 15, 2007, http://www.decanter.com/news/149578.html (accessed December 12, 2009).

Endnotes, Chapter 7

1. King James Version.
2. Paula Hook and Joe Heimlich, "A History of Packaging," Ohio State University Fact Sheet CDFS-133, Columbus, OH, http://ohioline.osu.edu/cd-fact/0133 .html (accessed December 12, 2009).
3. "Water, water everywhere," Container Recycling Institute report, 2007, http://www.container-recycling.org/assets/pdfs/reports/2007-waterwater.pdf (accessed December 12, 2009).
4. Personal communication from Benjamin Morse at Platts.com, December 16, 2008.
5. P..H. Gleick and H. Cooley, "Energy Implications of Bottled Water," *Environmental Research Letters* 4, doi:10.1088/1748-9326/4/1/014009 (2009), http://www.iop.org/EJ/article/1748-9326/4/1/014009/erl9_1_014009.pdf?request-id =c9869bfa-8642-463a-b930-afe1foe83cac (accessed November 2, 2009).
6. Steve Pardo, "Bottled water backlash: Cities, critics knock the high cost, waste," *Detroit News*, July 15, 2008.
7. Mike Schedler, "A PET Bottle recycling status report," *Resource Recycling*, February 2006, 2–4.
8. British Broadcasting Corporation, "Recycling around the world," television program, June 25, 2005, http://news.bbc.co.uk/2/hi/europe/4620041.stm (accessed December 12, 2009); see also "Plastics recovery reaches 50 percent in Europe by 2006," http://www.plastemart.com/upload/Literature/Plastics -recovery-reaches-50percent-in-Europe.asp (accessed December 12, 2009).
9. Kalyan Moitra, "Recycle Onus on PET Producers, Says PCB," *Economic Times of India*, June 27, 2003.
10. National Association for PET Container Resources (NAPCOR), 2004 Report on Post-Consumer PET Container Recycling Activity, Final Report, Sonoma, CA, http://www.napcor.com/PET/pet_reports.html (accessed December 12, 2009).
11. Coca-Cola Company, "Coca-Cola and National Recycling Coalition Launch Recycle Bin Grant Program," press release, September 26, 2007.
12. See, for example, this archived page on the Coca-Cola company website from February 2007: http://web.archive.org/web/20070205185315/www.thecocacola company.com/contactus/faq/environment.html (accessed December 12, 2009).
13. *Environmental Leader: Energy and Environmental News for Business* (website), "2nd UK Beverage Maker Claims 1st to Use 100% Recycled Plastic Bottle," September 27, 2007, http://www.environmentalleader.com/2007/09/27/2nd -uk-beverage-maker-claims-1st-to-use-100-recycled-plastic-bottle/ (accessed December 10, 2009).
14. Kenneth Marsh and Betty Bugusu, "Food packaging—Roles, materials, and environmental issues," *Journal of Food Science* 72, no. 3 (2007).
15. See Elizabeth Royte, "Corn plastic to the rescue," *Smithsonian Magazine*, August, 2000, http://www.smithsonianmagazine.com/issues/2006/august/pla .php (accessed December 12, 2009).

16. Institute for Local Self-Reliance, "Recycling Coalition Calls for Moratorium on PLA Bottles," press release, October 20, 2006, http://www.ilsr.org/columns/2006/102006.html (accessed December 12, 2009).

17. Primo Water Company, "Primo Launches More Environmentally Friendly Bottled Water in Time for Earth Day 2008," press release, April 7, 2008, http://www.primowater.com/news_pr_20080407_01.php (accessed December 12, 2009).

18. PLA World Congress, Congress brochure, 2008, http://www.pla-world-congress.com/brochure.pdf (accessed December 12, 2009).

19. Carleton University, Minutes of Joint Health and Safety Committee Meeting #142, January 25, 2006, Agenda Item 05-21 Drinking Water Fountains, http://www.carleton.ca/ehs/ehsjhsc/minutes/minutes142-25jan06.pdf (accessed December 12, 2009).

20. Allison Cross, "NDP accuses UBC of encouraging students to drink bottled water," *Vancouver Sun*, June 25, 2008, http://www2.canada.com/vancouversun/news/story.html?id=a5716191-5310-4588-9553-aa9387f9f919&k=93127 (accessed December 12, 2009).

21. Bottled Water Alliance, "Australia: Oh Bubbler, Where Art Thou?" Press release, January 16, 2009, http://www.bottledwateralliance.com.au/en/News%20and%20media/~/media/Files/BWA/Bubbler%20Project%20Release%2016-1-09.ashx (accessed December 12, 2009).

22. A. Ferguson, "The Mess on the Mall: Confusion reigns supreme on America's promenade," *The Weekly Standard*, August 15, 2005, http://www.weeklystandard.com/Content/Public/Articles/000/000/005/933yvhhs.asp (accessed October 22, 2009).

23. New Yorkers for Parks, "The Report Card on Parks 2007: An Independent Assessment of New York's Neighborhood Parks," 14, http://www.ny4p.org/index.php?option=com_docman&task=doc_download&gid=132 (accessed December 12, 2009).

Endnotes, Chapter 8

1. John Benson, "Pseudo Scientific Arguments in Advertising," *Advertising and Selling* 8 (February 23, 1927): 85. See n. 11

2. Dan Hurley, "Natural Causes: Death, Lies, and Politics in America's Vitamin and Herbal Supplement Industry," *Business Week*, January 8, 2007, http://www.businessweek.com/magazine/content/07_02/b4016109.htm?chan=search (accessed December 12, 2009).

3. For example, certain fatty acids found in some species of snakes contain eicosapentaenoic acid, which has anti-inflammatory properties. See R. A. Kunin, "Snake oil," *Western Journal of Medicine* 151, no. 2 (August 1989): 208, http://www.pubmedcentral.nih.gov/picrender.fcgi?artid=1026931&blobtype=pdf (accessed September 23, 2008).

4. As described by James Harvey Young in *The Medical Messiahs: A Social History of Healthy Quackery in Twentieth-Century America* (Princeton, NJ: Princeton University Press, 1967), 322–23. The first law giving authority of the Postal Service to issue fraud orders was 17 Stat. 322-323 (June 18, 1872).

5. In 1901, the Annual Report of the postmaster general (Washington, D.C.: U.S. Government Printing Office) refers to "quack medicines." (*Report of the Postmaster General*, 1901, 36).

6. 34 Stat. 768, Ch. 3914 Pure Food and Drugs Act of 1906.

7. *New York Times* editorial, "Guaranteed," July 2, 1906, 6.

8. United States Pure Food and Drugs Act of 1906 (34 Stat. 768), Section 8 as amended by the Act of August 23, 1912, c. 352, 37 Stat. 416.

9. Young, *The Medical Messiahs*, 115.

10. Ibid., 116, citing Roland Cole, "Standard Remedies," *Printers Ink* 122, no. 1 (February 1915): 27.

11. John Benson, "Pseudo Scientific Arguments in Advertising," *Advertising and Selling* 8 (Feb 23, 1927): 85. (Cited in Young, *The Medical Messiahs*, 146).

12. Young, *The Medical Messiahs*, 117.

13. William E. Humphrey, "Publishers and False Advertising," speech before the National Petroleum Association, September 17, 1926, FTC Speech File, cited by Young, *The Medical Messiahs*, 118.

14. H. A. Batten, "An Advertising Man Looks at Advertising," *Atlantic Monthly*, July 1932, 53.

15. P. Z. Myers, "Kabbalah Water? Pseudoscientific Hokum," *Pharyngula*, July 6, 2005, http://pharyngula.org/index/weblog/comments/kabbalah_water _pseudoscientific_hokum/ (accessed May 23, 2009).

16. Hado Water, http://www.hado-energie.nl/hado_water.php (accessed December 12, 2009).

17. Tools for Wellness, "Millennium Oxygen Water Cooler," http://www.toolsfor wellness.com/33801.html (accessed January 22, 2009).

18. Applied Ozone Systems, "Oxygen Deficiency Disease," http://www.applied ozone.com/oxygen_deficiency_disease.html (accessed January 24, 2009).

19. R. A. Berner, "Atmospheric oxygen over Phanerozoic time," *Proceedings of the National Academy of Sciences* 96, no. 20 (1999): 10955–957, http://www.pnas .org/content/96/20/10955.full. See also, C. Clairborne Ray, "Breathing Room," *New York Times*, http://www.nytimes.com/2008/03/04/science/04qna .html (accessed December 12, 2009).

20. O₂ Canada, "Superoxygenated Spring Water," http://www.ocanadawater.com/ oxygenatedwater.html (accessed March 17, 2009).

21. See, for example, Nancy Willmert, John P. Porcari, Carl Foster, Scott Dober-stein, and Glenn Brice, "The Effects of Oxygenated Water on Exercise Physiol-ogy during Incremental Exercise and Recovery," *Journal of Exercise Physiology* online 5, no. 4 (Nov 2002), http://faculty.css.edu/tboone2/asep/Porcari.pdf (accessed March 17, 2009); and C. A. Piantadosi, "Oxygenated water and ath-letic performance: Ergogenic claims for oxygenated water cannot be taken seri-ously," *British Journal of Sports Medicine* 40 (July 2006): 740–41.

22. N. B. Hampson, N. W. Pollock, and C. A. Piantadosi, "Oxygenated water and athletic performance," *JAMA* 290 (2003): 2408–09, http://jama.ama-assn.org/ cgi/content/full/290/18/2408-b (accessed March 17, 2009).

23. Georgia Institute of Technology, "Oxygenated water: Fad and fiction in one expensive burp," http://web.archive.org/web/20030816133251/www.gatech

.edu/news-room/archive/news_releases/sports-august2001.html (accessed March 17, 2009).

24. "FTC Charges Marketer of 'Vitamin O' with Making False Health Claims," FTC File No. 992 3107, Civil Action No. CS-99-0063-EFS, 15 March 1999, http://www.ftc.gov/opa/1999/03/rosecreek.shtm (accessed March 17, 2009).

25. Federal Trade Commission v. Rose Creek Health Products Inc., The Staff of Life Inc., and Donald L. Smyth. Complaint for Permanent Injunction and Other Equitable Relief, March 15, 1999, http://www.ftc.gov/os/1999/03/rosecreekcmp.htm (accessed December 7, 2008).

26. See http://www.ftc.gov/opa/2000/05/rosecreek2.shtm.

27. High Power Supplements, "Vitamin O," http://www.highpowersupplements.com/VitaminO.html?source=adwords (accessed November 9, 2007).

28. Shopwiki.com, "Rose Creek Vitamin 'O' Stabilized Oxygen," http://www.shopwiki.com/detail/d=Rose_Creek_Vitamin_%22O%22_Stabilized_Oxygen_4_oz/jumpToFirst=t/ (accessed January 22, 2009); see also the Yahoo! shopping sites under "Nutrition, Vitamins, and Supplements," Yahoo.com, http://shopping.yahoo.com/s:Nutrition,%20Vitamins%20&%20Supplements:4168-Brand= Rose%20Creek (accessed January 22, 2009).

29. Richard L. Cleland, Walter C. Gross, Laura D. Koss, Matthew Daynard, and Karen M. Muoio, "Weight-Loss Advertising: An Analysis of Current Trends," Federal Trade Commission, 2002, http://www.ftc.gov/bcp/reports/weightloss.pdf (accessed December 12, 2009).

30. For a listing of Federal Trade Commission Advertising Cases Involving Weight-Loss Products and Services, 1927–May 2003, see http://www.dietscam.org/reg/ ftclist.shtml (accessed December 12, 2009).

31. Dieta Formas, http://www.agualuso.pt/index.html?2 (accessed December 7, 2008).

32. eVamor, "About the eVamor product," http://www.evamor.com/about-the-product/about-the-product.php (accessed December 7, 2008).

33. Jana Skinny Water, Creative Enterprises Inc., 2005, http://web.archive.org/web/20050923220949/http://www.skinnywater.com/ (accessed December 12, 2009).

34. Healthy Weight Network, http://www.healthyweight.net/fraud1.html (accessed May 22, 2009).

35. Hilary E. MacGregor, "Health conscious embrace trendy water," Los Angeles Times, January 26, 2006, http://www.azcentral.com/health/wellness/articles/0126water.html (accessed December 12, 2009).

36. Max H. Pittler and Edzard Ernst, "Dietary supplements for body-weight reduction: a systematic review," The American Journal of Clinical Nutrition 79, no. 4 (2004): 529–36.

37. J. L. van de Haar, P. Y. Wielinga, A. J. W. Scheurink, and A. G. Nieuwenhuizen, "Comparison of the effects of three different (−)-hydroxycitric acid preparations on food intake in rats," Nutrition & Metabolism 2 (2005): 23, doi:10.1186/1743-7075-2-23, http://www.biomedcentral.com/content/pdf/1743-7075-2-23.pdf (accessed December 7, 2008); see also "Garcinia Cambogia: A Natural Weight Loss Supplement Ingredient," http://www.articlesbase.com/weight-loss-articles/garcinia-cambogia-a-natural-weight-loss

-supplement-ingredient-360968.html (accessed December 12, 2009).

38. Jon Swaine, "Weight loss water criticised by food watchdog," *The Telegraph*, August 11, 2008, http://www.telegraph.co.uk/news/uknews/2538530/Weight -loss-water-criticised-by-food-watchdog.html (accessed December 7, 2008).

39. See, for example, such claims listed in http://www.articlesbase.com/coffee -articles/the-difference-between-skinny-water-and-other-fitness-drinks-735145 .html (accessed December 13, 2009).

40. *Aquatechnology.net*, "A Review of Masaru Emoto's Functional Water Writings," http://www.aquatechnology.net/emoto.html (accessed 5 October 2008). See also Dr. Emoto's actual book, http://hado-energie.nl/TruthofHado.pdf (down-loaded January 25, 2009).

41. Stace Sharp, "Miraculous Messages from Water," http://www.wellnessgoods .com/messages.asp (accessed January 26, 2009).

42. Masaru Emoto, "Truth of Hado," published by PHP Kenkyuujyo, 1994, http://hado-energie.nl/TruthofHado.pdf (accessed October 5, 2008).

43. Quoted in Gustav von Bunge *Lehrbuch der Physiologie des Menschen*, 2nd ed. (Leipzig, Germany: Verlag von F. C. W. Vogel), 1901. Digitized November 28, 2007, http://books.google.com/books?id=jfgRAAAAYAAJ (accessed September 29, 2009).

44. Hado Water, "Dr. Emoto's Hexagonal Water," http://www.hado.net/indigo water/indigo_water.php (accessed December 12, 2009).

45. Royal Spring Water Inc., "World's First Commercial Agronifier Machine used to Transform Water into Structured Water, has been Installed, Tested and is Fully Operational at the Royal Spring Water Inc. Bottling Plant in Hereford, TX," press release, February 16, 2007, http://www.royalspringswater. com/pdf/Press%20Release%2002-16-2007.pdf (accessed February 28, 2007).

46. H$_2$Om: Water with Intention, "Our Infusion Process," http://www.h2om water.com/infusionprocess.html (accessed October 3, 2008).

47. Ibid.

48. Paul Adams, "Lamest Value-Added Products," *Wired* Magazine, May 9, 2007, http://www.wired.com/culture/lifestyle/multimedia/2007/05/gallery_value adding?slide=1&slideView=3 (accessed December 12, 2009).

49. Aquamanta company, "Aquamantra—Bottled Water Infused with Luck Gives Oscar Nominees the Edge," press release, February 21, 2007, from PRWeb Press Release Newswire, http://aquamantra.com/vg_images/news/AM_Oscars _2007.pdf (downloaded December 12, 2009).

50. Aquamantra, "What is Aquamantra?" http://aquamantra.com/site.php/spgs /read/what_is_aquamantra (accessed October 3, 2008).

51. Aquamantra, "How is our water created?" http://aquamantra.com/site.php/ spgs/read/taste_the_difference (accessed October 3, 2008).

52. Keith J. Petrie and Simon Wessely, "Getting Well from Water," *BMJ* 329, nos. 18–25 (December 2004): 1417–418, http://www.fmhs.auckland.ac.nz/som/ psychmed/petrie/_docs/2005_getting_well_from_water.pdf (downloaded December 13, 2009).

53. Dana Coffield, "Experts help wade through bottled-water choices," *Denver Post*, . June 14, 2005.

54. Dan Quattrone, "Doing Things With Words: Metaphysics (The Bad Kind)," blog, June 5, 2005, http://dtww.blogspot.com/2005/06/metaphysics-bad-kind .html (accessed December 13, 2009).

55. Zunami, "H$_2$O clusters," http://www.clusteredwateronline.com/H$_2$OClusters .html (accessed October 3, 2008).

56. Tim Elliott, "A Stiff Drink: Virginality, Minerality, or Gullibility," February 20, 2007, http://www.container-recycling.org/media/newsarticles/plastic/2007/2 -20-Australia-AStiffDrink.htm (accessed December 13, 2009).

57. Bottled Water Web, "Penta Water," http://www.bottledwaterweb.com/ bottlersdetail.do?k=64 (accessed May 25, 2009).

58. Penta Water, "Hydrate for Life," May 29, 2001, available at http://web .archive.org/web/20010625094505/www.hydrateforlife.com/what.shtml (accessed October 23, 2009).

59. Penta Water, "Research and Studies," available at http://web.archive.org/web/ 20021207223427/pentawater.com/research.shtml; see also: "Penta Water: Hydrate Your Life," http://web.archive.org/web/20021201031512/http ://penta water.com/.

60. Penta Water, "Penta Water: Taste and Feel the Difference," http://web. archive .org/web/20030523084442/http://pentawater.com/.

61. James Randi, "A Classic Case of Challenge, Acceptance, Stalling, Misrepresen- tation, and a Final Retreat: The Penta Water Case," http://www.randi .org/jr/08-24-01.html (accessed May 22, 2009).

62. James Randi, "A Classic Case of Challenge, Acceptance, Stalling, Misrepresen- tation, and a Final Retreat: The Penta Water Case," Penta Part 1 and 2, http:// www.randi.org/jr/08-24-01.html and http://www.randi.org/jr/08-31-01.html (accessed December 13, 2009).

63. For a summary of the exchanges between Randi and Holloway, see http://www .randi.org/jr/08-24-01.html and http://www.randi.org/jr/08-31-01.html (accessed December 13, 2009).

64. Advertising Standards Authority, "Against Penta UK," ASA British Penta Water Adjudication, http://www.asa.org.uk/asa/adjudications/non_broadcast/ Adjudication+Details.htm?Adjudication_id=39409 (accessed December 13, 2009).

65. Bottled Water Web, "Penta Water," http://www.bottledwaterweb.com/ bottlersdetail.do?k=64 (accessed November 8, 2007).

66. Penta Water, "Research and Studies," http://www.pentawater.com/research .shtml#physical (accessed February 12, 2008), now available at http://web .archive.org/web/20080212130932/ http://www.pentawater.com/research .shtml.

67. Penta Water, "What is Penta," http://www.pentawater.com/_pw/pentafacts .php?sub=1&item=4 (accessed March 6, 2009).

Endnotes, Chapter 9

1. Newsletter of the Fifth Episcopal District Women's Missionary Society of the African Methodist Episcopal Church, http://www.nccecojustice.org/down loads/Ecological_Justice_Special_Edition.pdf (accessed January 25, 2008).

2. The Kabbalah Centre International, "What is Kabbalah?" http://www .kabbalah.com/01.php (accessed January 25, 2009).

3. Olivia Barker, "Madonna has faith on a string," *USA Today*, May 25, 2004, http://www.usatoday.com/life/lifestyle/2004-05-25-kabbalah-main_x.htm (accessed December 12, 2009).

4. Ibid.

5. *San Francisco Chronicle*, "The Daily Dish: Madonna tour fueled by Kabbalah water," May 25, 2006, http://www.sfgate.com/cgi-bin/blogs/sfgate/detail?blog id=7&entry_id=5513 (accessed December 12, 2009).

6. The Kabbalah Centre International, "Kabbalah Water," http://www.kabbalah water.com (accessed October 5, 2008).

7. Stace Sharp, "Miraculous Messages from Water: How Water Reflects Our Consciousness," http://www.wellnessgoods.com/messages.asp (accessed October 5, 2008).

8. Ben Wasserstein, "Department of Labor," *In Touch* and *Slate*, August 19, 2005, http://www.slate.com/id/2124696/.

9. Reporting by Jennifer Wulff, Michael Fleeman, Lycia Naff, Alison Singh Gee, and Nicholas White in Los Angeles, Samantha McIntyre in New York City, *People Magazine*, October 3, 2005.

10. Art Levine, "The Accidental Kabbalist," *City Link Magazine*, January 24, 2001, http://www.rickross.com/reference/kabbalah/kabbalah26.html (accessed May 22, 2009); see also Richard Batholomew, "Mystic Water and Katherine Harris," *Bartholomew's Notes on Religion* (website), July 5, 2005, http://barthsnotes .wordpress.com/2005/07/07/mystic-water-and-katherine-harris/ (accessed May 22, 2009).

11. Jim Stratton, "'Celestial Drops' no cure for canker; Florida researched the use of water, possibly mystically blessed, to cure the disease," *Orlando Sentinel*, July 5, 2005, http://www.orlandosentinel.com/business/orl-aseccanker05070505 jul05,0,3793083.story?page=1&coll=orl-home-headlines (accessed May 22, 2009).

12. The Safe Drinking Water Trust, "Can Water Systems Compete with Heaven?" January 10, 2007, http://www.watertrust.org/news_article.asp?nID=67; see also Cheryl Winkelman, *Inside Bay Area*, www.insidebayarea.com/argus/ localnews/ci_4970271.

13. Holy Spring Water website, http://www.holywater.biz/main.html (accessed December 12, 2009).

14. Liquid Salvation, http://www.liquidsalvation.com (accessed August 10, 2008).

15. Rebecca U. Cho, "Groups hope to make bottled water a moral issue," Religion New Service, December 19, 2006, http://www.faithinpubliclife.org/content/ news/2006/12/groups_hope_to_make_bottled_wa.html (accessed December 12, 2009).

16. Ibid.

17. Ibid.

18. Joel Connelly, "Episcopal Bishops Say Don't Go Near the (Bottled) Water," *Seattle Post-Intelligencer*, May 5, 2009, http://www.virtueonline.org/portal/ modules/news/article.php?storyid=10382 (accessed May 22, 2009).

19. Father Robert A. Sirico, "Blessing the Waters," *National Catholic Register*, February 25–March 3, 2007.

Endnotes, Chapter 10

1. J. Colson, "Bottled water backlash?" *The Aspen Times*, August 14, 2007.
2. M. J. Credeur and T. Mulier, "Nestlé loses sales as Alice Waters bans bottled water," Bloomberg News, January 22, 2008, http://www.bloomberg.com/apps/news?pid=20601109&sid=aHgE5mVQHAVM (accessed March 2, 2008).
3. D. McLaren, "Canada: Time to turn back to the tap?" *Globe and Mail* (Toronto), April 22, 2008.
4. Canadean (Basingstoke, England), "Bottled Water Growth Slows as Consumers Turn on the Tap: Latest Global Beverage Forecasts from Canadean," March 18, 2009, http://www.canadean.com/Portals/0/news/canadean_press_releases/pdf/general/Global%20Beverage%20Forecasts%20press%20orelease.pdf (accessed December 12, 2009).
5. "French bottled water sales slipping as consumers turn to tapwater—Report," AFX News Limited, March 29, 2007.
6. M. Hickman, "Bottled water sales starting to run dry," *The Independent*, March 23, 2009, http://www.independent.co.uk/environment/green-living/bottled-water-sales-starting-to-run-dry-1651724.html (accessed September 23, 2009).
7. Richard Girard, "Bottled Water Industry Faces Downward Spiral," *Alternet*, March 11, 2009, http://www.alternet.org/workplace/130920/bottled_water_industy_faces_downward_spiral/?page=entire (accessed August 12, 2009).
8. Tom Lauria, "Bottled Water Market Share Volume Increased in 2008," International Bottled Water Association, April 1, 2009, http://www.bottled water.org/news/bottled-water-market-share-volume-increased-2008 (accessed December 13, 2009).
9. Canadian Broadcasting Corporation News, "Drop in bottled water sales encourages activists," February 19, 2009, http://www.cbc.ca/consumer/story/2009/ 02/19/nestle-water.html (accessed May 28, 2009); see also "Inside the Bottle" campaign, "2008 Bottled Water Profits Down: Bottled Water Bans Up," press release, February 19, 2009, http://www.insidethe bottle.org/2008-bottled-water-profits-down-bottled-water-bans (accessed May 28, 2009).
10. AFP (Agence France-Presse), "Let them drink tap-water: Paris fights back against the bottle," March 22, 2005.
11. Charles Bremner, "Paris Water Wars," *Times* (London), January 19, 2007, http://timescorrespondents.typepad.com/charles_bremner/2007/01/french_advertis.html#more (accessed May 28, 2009).
12. Stuart Elliott, "An honor for creativity fuels odes to tap water," *New York Times*, November 17, 2006.
13. P. McGreevy, "Mayor reasserts ban on bottled-water purchases," *Los Angeles Times*, January 6, 2006.
14. Bethan Dorsett, "£35,000 cap on bottled water: A Council is planning to stop supplying mineral water to staff in a bid to save money," *Manchester Evening News*, January 27, 2007, http://www.manchestereveningnews.co.uk/news/s/

234/234436_35000_cap_on_bottled_water.html (accessed October 10, 2009).

15. Andrea Weigl, "Dissension, drop by drop: Bottled water earns wrath of environmentalists. But the issues aren't cut and dried," *News and Observer* (Salt Lake City), April 16, 2008, www.newsobserver.com/105/v-print/story/1038560. html (accessed January 10, 2009).

16. "Seattle bans city purchases of bottled water," *WaterTech* Online, March 19, 2008.

17. Michelle Durand, "County says bottled water idea all wet," *Daily Journal* (San Mateo County, CA), May 1, 2009, http://www.smdailyjournal.com/article_preview.php?id=109660 (accessed May 26, 2009).

18. Susan Haigh, "With budgets tapped, governors eye cost of water," *Ventura County Star* (CA), February 13, 2009, http://www.venturacountystar.com/news/2009/feb/13/with-budgets-tapped-governors-eye-cost-of-water/ (accessed May 28, 2009).

19. Memorandum of Decision and Judgment, June 1, 2009, Circuit Court of Cook County, Illinois, No 08-CH-396: American Beverage Association, International Bottled Water Association, Illinois Retail Merchants Association, and Illinois Food Retailers Association v. City of Chicago.

20. Jason Ericson, "'Holding the water for us to see it:' New artist-designed outdoor drinking fountains in Minneapolis," *Twin Cities Daily Planet* (Minneapolis, MN), July 15, 2008, http://www.tcdailyplanet.net/article/2008/06/24/holding-water-us-see-it-new-artist-designed-outdoor-drinking-fountains-minneapolis (accessed May 28, 2009).

21. Pippa Crerar, "Boris wants fountains to replace bottles," *Evening Standard* (London), June 10, 2008, http://www.thisislondon.co.uk/standard-mayor/article23492331-details/Boris+wants+fountains+to+replace+bottles/article.do (accessed June 4, 2009).

22. G. Ruhe, "School water fountains to prevent obesity," *New York Times* Well Blog, March 30, 2009.

23. Michelle Locke, "Chez Panisse among restaurants leading bottled water backlash," *Fresno Bee*, March 28, 2007.

24. Incanto Restaurant, http://www.incanto.biz/why.html (accessed August 22, 2008).

25. M. J. Credeur and T. Mulier, "Nestlé loses sales as Alice Waters bans bottled water," Bloomberg News, http://www.bloomberg.com/apps/news?pid=20601109&refer=news&sid=aHgE5mVQHAVM (accessed March 2, 2008).

26. A. Weigl, "Dissension, drop by drop," *News and Observer* (Toronto), April 18, 2008, www.newsobserver.com/105/v-print/story/1038560.html.

27. *FineWaters.com*, "Tap water only at fine restaurants?" *Water Connoisseur*, April 1, 2007, http://www.finewaters.com/Newsletter/The_Water_Connoisseur_Archive/Tap_Water_Only_at_Fine_Restaurants.asp (accessed December 12, 2009).

28. Barbara Whitaker, "For Town, Water Is a Fighting Word," *New York Times*, March 23, 2003, http://query.nytimes.com/gst/fullpage.html?res=9C07E6D81630F930A15750C0A9659C8B63 (accessed May 28, 2009).

29. Anne Wallace, "Cold Mountain Spring," *The Green Guide* 101, March/April 2004 (downloaded July 27, 2007); see also Kenneth Miller, "An Idyll Interrupted," *Los Angeles Times Magazine*, August 1, 2004.

30. "Fujiaqua bottled water was not licensed," *Yomiuri Shimbun* (Japan), December 31, 2006.

31. Kevin Miller, "H$_2$O takes new tack against big bottlers," *Bangor Daily News*, March 2, 2007, http://www.accessmylibrary.com/article-1G1-160040667/h2o -takes-new-tack.html (accessed December 12, 2009).

32. Glen Martin, "Bottled water war heats up election," *San Francisco Chronicle*, November 5, 2006, http://www.sfgate.com/cgi-bin/article/article?f=/c/a/ 2006/11/05/BAGR8M6ID11.DTL (accessed December 12, 2009).

33. Diane Lowe, "Update on Nestlé Bottling Plant Threatening Mount Shasta's Aquifer," Mount Shasta Bioregional Center, August 21, 2006, http://www .indybay.org/newsitems/2006/08/21/18299272.php.

34. ECONorthwest (Eugene, OR), "The Potential Economic Effects of the Proposed Water Bottling Facility in McCloud," October 2007, http://www .caltrout.org/docs/ECONRpt.pdf (accessed March 18, 2009).

35. R. S. Rappold, "Water-permit application by Nestlé taps wellspring of conflict in community," *The Colorado Springs Gazette*, May 1, 2009, http://www .gazette.com/articles/salida-52835-chaffee-save.html (accessed December 12, 2009).

36. Andrea Weigl, Corporate Accountability International, "Bottled water earns wrath of environmentalists," *Raleigh News and Observer*, http://www.stop corporateabuse.org/raleigh-news-observer-dissention-drop-drop (accessed December 12, 2009).

37. *The Scotsman*, "Bottled Water 'Damages Environment' Especially with a 10K Mile Delivery," November 10, 2004, http://www.iema.net/news/envnews ?aid=4894j (accessed May 28, 2009).

38. M. Wainwright, "Leeds students ban bottled water," *Guardian* (London), December 16, 2008.

39. Sophie Haydock, "Ban bottled water," *Guardian*, December 20, 2008, http://www.guardian.co.uk/commentisfree/2008/dec/20/bottled-water -ban-leeds (accessed December 12, 2009).

40. Inside the Bottle, "Students at McGill vote to end the sale and distribution of bottled water," February 18, 2009, http://www.insidethebottle.org/students -mcgill-vote-end-sale-and-distribution-bottled-water (accessed May 28, 2009); see also, Joe Cressy, "Celebrating the beginning of the end of bottled water in Canada," Rabble News, http://rabble.ca/news/2009/12/celebrating-beginning -end-bottled-water-canada (accessed December 12, 2009).

41. IBWA, "IBWA Media Relations 2006 and 2007" (as of September 1, 2007), memo prepared for the IBWA Communications Committee.

42. IBWA, "Corporate Accountability International Campaign Confuses Customers and Provides Bottled Water Misinformation," press release, October 10, 2007, http://www.waterwebster.com/IBWAchallengesCorporateAccount abilityInternationalOct.102007.htm (accessed December 12, 2009).

43. J. Wiggins, "UK: Bottlers of water try to turn off the tap," *Financial Times*,

November 25, 2008, http://us.ft.com/ftgateway/superpage.ft?news_id=fto
112320081306183798 (accessed May 28, 2009).

44. J. Colson, "Bottled water backlash?" *Aspen Times*, August 14, 2007.

45. C. Morgan, "Bottled water firm steamed about Miami-Dade water ads," *Miami Herald*, October 13, 2008.

46. Barry Massey, "More tax free coffee, water under Senate bill," Associated Press, February 28, 2007.

47. *The Business Review* (Albany, New York), "Nestlé Waters sues NY over bottle bill," May 19, 2009, http://albany.bizjournals.com/albany/stories/2009/05/18/daily19.html (accessed December 12, 2009).

Endnotes, Chapter 11

1. Marketwire, "Bottled Water Saves the World," August 24, 2007, http://www.marketwire.com/mw/release.do?id=764027&sourceType=3 (accessed December 14, 2009).

2. Poland Spring Company, "Eco-shape: A Better Bottle for You and Our Environment," advertisement, http://www.polandspring.com/DoingOurPart/EcoShapeBottle.aspx (accessed December 14, 2009).

3. Remarks of E. Neville Isdell, Chairman and CEO of the Coca-Cola Company, at the WWF Annual Conference, Beijing, China, June 5, 2007, The Coca-Cola Company Press Center, http://www.thecoca-colacompany.com/presscenter/viewpoints_isdell_wwf.html (accessed December 14, 2009).

4. The Coca-Cola Company Press Center, "Coca-Cola, URRC open world's largest plastic bottle-to-bottle recycling plant," press release, January 14, 2009, http://www.thecoca-colacompany.com/presscenter/nr_20090114_bottle-to-bottle_recycling.html (accessed September 28, 2009).

5. Marketwire, "Bottled Water Saves the World," August 24, 2007, http://www.marketwire.com/mw/release.do?id=764027&sourceType=3 (accessed December 14, 2009).

6. Belu Water advertisement, http://www.belu.org/ (accessed December 14, 2009).

7. Laura Devlin, "Campaigner Hailed Great Briton," *Eastern Daily Press*, May 23, 2007, http://new.edp24.co.uk/content/news/story.aspx?brand=EDPOnline&category=News&tBrand=EDPOnline&Category=news&itemid=NOED22%20May%202007%2022%3A20%3A13%3A170 (accessed December 14, 2009).

8. FoodBev Media, "One Water Founder Honored at UK Business Awards," November 21, 2008, http://water.foodbev.com/ArticleDetail.aspx?contentId=1793 (accessed May 27, 2009).

9. NameWire, "Neau: A Novel Product Name and Product Idea," Strategic Name Development, Inc., October 6, 2005, http://www.namedevelopment.com/blog/archives/2005/10/neau_a_novel_product_name_and_product_idea.html (accessed January 4, 2006).

10. *Marketplace*, "2008's greenwashes of the year," American Public Media, http://www.publicradio.org/columns/sustainability/greenwash/2008/12/2008s_greenwashes_of_the_year.html (accessed December 14, 2009).

11. See, for example, The Campaign to End Bottled Water, http://www.endbottled water.com/ (accessed December 14, 2009), or the Polaris Institute's "Inside the Bottle" Campaign, http://www.polarisinstitute.org/water (accessed December 14, 2009), or Corporate Accountability International's Think Outside the Bottle Campaign, http://www.stopcorporateabuse.org/think-outside-bottle (accessed December 14, 2009).

Endnotes, Chapter 12

1. Steve Conner, "Report attacks environmental costs of dams," *Independent* (London), November 17, 2000, http://www.independent.co.uk/environment/report -attacks-environmental-cost-of-dams-621924.html (accessed December 13, 2009).
2. P. H. Gleick, "Global Freshwater Resources: Soft-Path Solutions for the 21st Century," *Science* 302 (November 2003): 1524–528.

Index

Figures/photos/illustrations are indicated by a " f."

Abbey, Edward, 63
Acton Institute, 140
advertising
    art of, 109–110
    ASA and, 129–130
    consumer protection agencies and, 116, 179
    expansion of, 112
    fear used in, 6–7
    Fiji, 14f
    Great Depression and, 113
    history regarding, 110–113
    of miracle cure, 113–114
    NBBB and, 112–113
    regulation of, 111–113, 116, 179
    slogans, 110
    snake oil and, 110–111
    taste influenced by, 82
    voluntary code of, 7–8
Advertising Standards Authority (ASA),
    129–130
aluminum, 90
American Water Works Association,
    10–11
Anderson, Rocky, 149
Aquafina, 7, 56, 59, 80, 145
Aquaid Ltd., 168
Aquamantra, 125–126
aqueducts, 18
"arctic," on label, 56–57
Arrowhead Spring Water, 52, 53–54, 56,
    65, 94, 96, 157
Arrowhead Spring Water Cabazon plant
    bottles made in, 71–72
    cleanliness of, 71
    description of, 64–65
    history concerning, 65
        source of water for, 65–66
        tour of, 71–72
        traveling to, 63–64
artesian water, 55
ASA. See Advertising Standards Authority
Athena Bottled Water, 168

Back to the Tap movement, 158
bacteria. See cholera; coliform bacteria
Barnum, P.T., 20
Barrington, New Hampshire, 74–75
Bastianich, Joseph, 153
Batali, Mario, 153
Batten, H.A., 113
beer, 21, 22
Bell, Peter, 85
Belu Water, 168
Benson, John, 109, 112
Berg, Yehuda, 134
Berkeley recycling system, 97–99
bisphenol A (BPA), 91
Black, Paul, 154–155
bottled water. See also advertising; contain-
        ers; convenience, cost of; ethical bot-
        tled water; future; industry;
        International Bottled Water Associa-
        tion; label; oxygen water; plastic bot-
        tle; polyethylene terephthalate; recalls;
        recycling; regulation; revolts; selling
        bottled water; taste; testing; weight-
        loss scams; specific label; specific regula-
        tory agency
    big numbers regarding, xi
    broader context concerning, x, xiii
    ethical issues regarding, xii
    pervasiveness of, 3, 5–6
    reasons for buying, xi–xii
    thousand a second and, x
Bowerman, Susan, 123
BPA. See bisphenol A

Bradford, William, 21
Bradley, Thomas, 149
Brett, Allen, 149
Brita, 10–11
Brod, Avrohom, 137
Bulcke, Paul, 146

Cabazon, 64, 65. *See also* Arrowhead
    Spring Water Cabazon plant
California
    legislation, 59–60
    McCloud, 156–157
Canadian Bottled Water Association, 145
Cardin, Pierre, 147
Carmichael, Cassandra, 139
CEI. *See* Competitive Enterprise Institute
Celestial Drops, 136
Central Park, 17, 20–21, 106
Chez Panisse, 153
Chilibeck, Kori, 163, 167
China, 69, 99
chlorination, 28f, 29
cholera
    bacteria causing, 25
    early efforts to understand, 23
    European/American waves of, 22–23
    Snow and, 24–25, 24f
Ciaccia, Julius, 15, 16
citrus canker, 136
Claridge's, 85
Clarke, Jeremy, 160
Clean Water Act (1972), 29
Cleveland, 29
    burning river in, 16
    Fiji ad and, 15, 16–17
    water quality in, 16–17
    water system in, 15
climate change, 174
clustered water. *See also* Penta Water
    claims surrounding, 124–126
    Emoto and, 124
    origins of, 123–124
    types of, 125–126
CNN list. *See* 101 Dumbest Moment in
    Business
Coca-Cola
    ethical bottled water efforts of, 164–165
    PlantBottle™ of, 105

recycling, 102
San Leandro plant of, 79–80
tap water and, 9–10
Cochran, Edward, 17
Code of Hammurabi, 173
coffee taste, 82
coliform bacteria
    bottled water regulation of, 38–39
    European regulation of, 39
    tap water regulation of, 37–38
Colorado, 157
commodity, water as private/public, 8–9
competition argument, 11–12
Competitive Enterprise Institute (CEI), 8, 9
consumer protection, 116, 117, 179
containers
    aluminum regarding, 90
    early, 88
    glass, 89
    improvements in, 89
    PET, 90–93
    recycling codes for, 89f
    safety of plastic, 90–91
contamination. *See also* pollution
    outside US, 49
    regulation and, 43–44
    types of, 47
convenience, cost of
    energy, 94–95
    environmental, 95–105
    garbage/landfill, 95–96
    incineration and, 103
    lightweighting and, 102–103
    public water and, 105–107
    questions surrounding, 93–94
    recycling and, 96–102
    tap water, 95
Cooley, Heather, 95
Corporate Accountability International
    IBWA countering, 159
    on regulations/standards, 33, 36
    Think Outside the Bottle campaign of,
      158
cost of convenience. *See* convenience,
    cost of
Coyle, Mary Ann, 140
crickets, 47
Crook, James King, 83

Cryptosporidium, 76–78
Cutler, David, 29
Cuyahoga River, 16, 29

Dasani, 9, 56, 79–80, 105, 110
Daughters of Charity, 139–140
Dearnley, Ashley, 149
Dee, Jon, 106
Dege, Nick, 65
deposit laws, 100–101
desert ecosystems, 66
diarrheal deaths, 28f
Dickens, Charles, Jr., 19
Dickson, James Tennant, 87, 88
Dingell, John, 43
disease, water-related
    alcohol and, 22
    cholera, 22–25
    federal agencies preventing, 29–30
    filtration preventing, 26
    history concerning, 21–25
    hydrologic cycle preventing, 25
    purification preventing, 26–29, 28f
    sterilization preventing, 27
Dorn, Nathaniel, 2–3
Doss, Joe, 11, 143
Drinking Water Research Foundation
    (DWRF)
    background, 73
    groundwater impact paper by, 72–73
    paper flaws, 73–74
DWRF. See Drinking Water Research
    Foundation

Earth Water, 167, 169
eaunologie, 84–85
Ecology Center, Berkeley, 97–98
Eco-shape® bottle, 164
Emoto, Masaru, 117, 124, 134, 135
energy costs, 94–95
"Enjoy Bottled Water" project, 9
environment
    cost of convenience regarding, 95–105
    friendly bottle, 103–105
    future reforms regarding, 179–180
Environmental Protection Agency (EPA)
    coliform regulation and, 37–38
    establishment of, 29

regulation, bottled water, and, 34–39
EPA. See Environmental Protection Agency
Erie, Lake, 29
    cleaning-up of, 16–17
    delivery of water from, 15
    pollution of, 16
ethical bottled water
    Belu Water, 168
    Earth Water, 167, 169
    Ethos Water, 165–167
    greenwashing and, 170
    issues, xii
    large producer efforts toward, 163–165
    lightweighting and, 164
    Neau water bottles and, 169–170
    One Water, 168–169
Ethos Water
    early development of, 165–166
    early growth of, 166–167
    Omidyars/Starbucks and, 167
    overview of, 169
    premise of, 166
    recall, 45–46
Europe
    cholera waves in, 22–23
    coliform bacteria and, 39
    label requirements in, 54, 59, 61t
"excessive," on label, 42

FDA. See Food and Drug Administration
fear, of tap water, 6–8, 17, 30–31
Federal Food and Drug and Cosmetic Act
    (FFDCA), 54
Federal Trade Commission (FTC)
    consumer protection and, 116, 117
    oxygen water and, 120–121
    weight-loss claims and, 121–122
Ferguson, Andrew, 106
FFDCA. See Federal Food and Drug and
    Cosmetic Act
Field, Moses, 20
Fiji
    advertisement, 14f
    Cleveland and, 15, 16–17
    greenwashing and, 170
    101 Dumbest Moment in Business
        and, 17
    quality of, 16–17

filtration, types of, 26
First Water Age, x, 172
Florida
    building code, 2
    Nestlé and, 160
    UCF football stadium fountains and, 1–3
Food and Drug Administration (FDA)
    coliform and, 38–39
    future regulation and, 178–179
    label reform and, 61, 189n15
    label requirements, 53–54, 58–59, 58f
    nutrition label, 58–59, 58f
    pathogenic organisms and, 76
    recalls and, 43–48
    regulation, bottled water, and, 34–39
    spring water designation, 72
    testing bottled water, 39–43
fossil ground water, 68–69
fountains. See water fountains
France, 147–148
Frank Water, 168
FTC. See Federal Trade Commission
Fujiaqua Company, 156
future
    hard path vision of, x–xi, 175–177
    industry reforms and, 178–180
    soft path vision of, xi, 174–175,
        177–178

GAO. See General Accounting Office
garbage, 95–96
General Accounting Office (GAO), 42
Germann, Brian, 136–137
Get Your Fill campaign, 148
Girard, Richard, 146
"glacier," on label, 57
glass bottles, 89
Glennon, Robert, 69
Google, 3, 143
Goose, Duncan, 168–169
Great Depression, 113
Greek water fountains, 18
green water. See ethical bottled water
Greenblat, Jonathan, 165, 166–167
greenwashing, 170
Grégoire, Renaud, 85
ground water. See also spring water
    Barrington, New Hampshire, 74–75

community concerns regarding, 72
deep fossil, 68–69
DWRF paper on, 72–74
Maricopa County, Arizona, 75
Ogallala aquifer and, 69–70
pathogenic organisms and, 76–78
problems with, 69–70
Sanctuary Springs, Michigan, 75
Standards of Identity and, 55
types of, 67–68

H2O for ME, 156
H2Om, 125
hard path vision, x–xi, 175–177
Hardoon, Abe, 136
Harms, Al, 2
Harris, Katherine, 136
Haydock, Sophie, 158
headlines, tap water, 30–31
Heston, Grant, 2
Hexagonal Indigo Water, 124
Hitt, John, 2
Holloway, William, 127, 129
Holy Drinking Water, 136–137
Holy Spring Water, 137–138
Howard, Brian, 51
Hubbard, L. Ron, 132
Humphrey, William E., 113
hydrologic cycle, 25, 67
hydroxycitric acid, 123

IBWA. See International Bottled Water
    Association
Idyllwild, 154–155
incineration, 103
industry
    competition argument of, 11–12
    contradictions in, 4
    groundwater impact and, 72–74
    growth of, 4–5
    on recycling, 96–97
    reforms needed in, 178–180
    self defense by, xii–xiii, 159–161
    shortcomings of, xiii
    US sales, 5, 5f
International Bottled Water Association
    (IBWA)
    annual convention, 8

California legislation and, 60
DWRF paper and, 73
on recycling, 96–97
on regulations/standards, 33
self defense by, 159
voluntary code of advertising, 7–8
Ireland, 49

Jana Skinny Water, 122–123
Jeffrey, Kim E., 35–36, 87, 91–92
Jennings, Bret, 153
Johnson, Benhu, 15
Johnson, Boris, 151

Kabbalah
    Celestial Drops and, 136
    commercial bent of, 133
    as cult, 132–133
    described, 132
    Harris and, 136
    Madonna as follower of, 133
    Spears as follower of, 135
Kabbalah Water
    claims for, 133, 134–135
    Madonna as user of, 133
    religion and, 132–135
    as spray, 133
    website for, 134
Kämtz, Ludwig Friedrich, 124
Kay, Stephen, 11
Knuttgen, Howard, 120
Koch, Robert, 25
Konikow, Leonard, 69
Kossa-Rienzi, Mike, 153
Kurst, Kyle, 65

label
    "arctic" on, 56–57
    California legislation and, 59–60
    European requirements, 54, 59, 61t
    "excessive" on, 42
    FDA and, 53–54, 58–59, 58f, 61,
        190n15
    future reforms for, 179
    "glacier" on, 57
    ideal information for, 53
    municipal water supply and, 56
    naming abuses on, 56–58

nutrition, 58–59, 58f
    reform of, 61, 190n15
    requirements, 53–54, 58–59, 58f
    source confusion and, 54, 56–58, 57t
    Standards of Identity, 54, 55
landfill, 95–96
Lapidus, Deborah, 158
Laporte, Dominique, 85
Lauria, Tom, 146
Lawless, Harry T., 83
Lawrence, Larry, 65
Leopold, King of Belgium, 21–22
lightweighting, 102–103, 164
Lim, Juyun, 83
Liquid Salvation, 138, 139f
Lombardi, Eric, 105
London, 3–4, 18–19
Los Angeles, 149

Madonna (pop icon), 133
Madureira, Franck, 147
Mandela, Nelson, 171
Maricopa County, Arizona, 75
Massachusetts 1785 legislation, 34, 35f
materials recovery facility (MRF), 99
McCloud, California, 156–157
McOmber, Marty, 150
Meagher, Virginia, 137
Metropolitan Free Drinking Fountain Asso-
    ciation, 18–19
Miller, Grant, 29
Mindel, Larry, 152
mineral water
    Standards of Identity and, 55
    taste regarding, 83
    website devoted to, 84
minerals
    Dasani and, 80
    taste and, 83–84
Mohave Desert, 63–64
Moorman, J.J., 83
Morongo Indian casino, 64
Morrison, Robert S., 7
MRF. See materials recovery facility
municipal water supply. See also tap water
    Dasani created from, 79–80
    future reforms for, 178
    label regarding, 56

Paris and, 147–148
spring water compared with, 75–76
taste tests with, 81
Myers, P.Z., 114–115

naming abuses, 56–58
National Better Business Bureau (NBBB),
    112–113
National Coalition of American Nuns, 140
National Council of Churches, 139
Natural Hydration Council, 160
NatureWorks, 104, 105
Naughton, Michelle, 56
NBBB. *See* National Better Business Bureau
Neau water bottles, 169–170
Nestlé Waters North America. *See also*
    Arrowhead Spring Water Cabazon
    plant
    acquisition of Cabazon facility, 65
    Eco-shape® bottle of, 164
    fights against, 156–157
    Florida fight by, 160
    New York State fight by, 161
    Poland Spring and, 51, 52–53
Netherlands, 49
New York City
    Get Your Fill campaign, 148
    tap water, 17–18, 25–26, 148
    using clean water sources, 25–26
    water fountains, 20–21
New York State, 161
Newman, Randy, 16
Newsom, Gavin, 149
Nielson, J. Christopher, 17
Nika Bottled Water, 168
nutrition label, 58–59, 58f

Obama, Barack, 43
Ogallala aquifer, 69–70
Okakura, Kakuzo, 63
Olin, Nelly, 148
Omidyar Network, 167
101 Dumbest Moment in Business (CNN
    list), 17
One Water, 168–169
oxygen water
    claims, 118–119
    FTC and, 120–121

science regarding, 119–120

Pacini, Filippo, 25
Paget, Reed, 168
Paris, 19, 147–148
pathogenic organisms, 76–78
Paul, Heidi, 65
PC. *See* polycarbonate
Penn and Teller, 85–86
Penta Water
    ASA challenging, 129–130
    claims of, 127–128, 130
    overview of, 126–127
    Randi challenging, 128–129
PepsiCo, 102, 164
Perrier recall, 46–47
PET. *See* polyethylene terephthalate
Pietsch, Daniel, 155
Pilgrims, 21–22
pixie dust, 80
PLA. *See* polylactic acid
PlantBottle™, 105
plastic bottle
    discovery leading to, 87–88
    energy costs of, 94–95
    environmentally friendly, 104–105
    incineration, 103
    lightweighting, 102–103, 164
    making of, 92–93
    PET, 90–93
    safety of, 90–91
Poland Spring
    history of, 51–52
    lawsuits regarding, 52
    Nestlé and, 51, 52–53
    sources of, 51, 53
Polaris Institue, 146
pollution
    federal agencies preventing, 29–30
    headlines regarding, 30–31
    history concerning, 21–25
    hydrologic cycle preventing, 25
    industrial/sewage dumping and, 26
    Lake Erie, 16
polycarbonate (PC), 91, 92
polyethylene terephthalate (PET)
    bottle, 90–93
    discovery of, 88

energy costs of, 94–95
garbage/landfill and, 95–96
lightweighting of, 102–103, 164
making bottles out of, 92–93
PLA compared to, 104
preforms, 92, 93f
recycling codes, 89f
recycling of, 97–102, 164–165
safety of, 90–91
polylactic acid (PLA), 104–105
polystyrene, 90–91
polyvinyl chloride (PVC), 90, 97
PRC. See Presbyterians for Restoring Creation
preforms, PET, 92, 93f
Presbyterians for Restoring Creation (PRC), 138
private wells, 185n13
pseudoscience
    clustered water, 123–126
    debunkers of, 114–115
    oxygen water, 118–121
    Penta Water, 126–130
    weight-loss scams, 121–123
public water
    convenience, cost of, and, 105–107
    disappearance of, 3, 171–172
    history regarding, 3–4
    saving system of, 171–172
Pure Food and Drugs Act, 111
purification
    filtration for, 26
    imitating nature, 27
    public health improvements via, 28–29, 28f
    sterilization methods for, 27
purified water, 55
PVC. See polyvinyl chloride

Randi, James, 115, 124, 128–129
Ransome, Kathleen, 7
recalls
    classes of, 44–45
    contaminants listed in, 47
    crickets and, 47
    FDA and, 43–48
    information on, 45–46
    notification of, 48

Perrier, 46–47
recycling
    Berkeley's system of, 97–99
    bottle recycled content and, 101–102
    bottled water industry on, 96–97
    Coca-Cola/PepsiCo and, 102
    codes, 89f
    deposit laws, 100–101
    Ecology Center, 97–98
    economics of, 99–100
    of PET, 97–102, 164–165
    rates, 97
    repackaging regarding, 99
regulation
    of advertising, 111–113, 116, 179
    coliform bacteria and, 37–39
    conflicting claims and, 35–36
    contamination, 43–44
    EPA/FDA and, 34–35, 36–38
    European, 39
    "excessive" label and, 42
    future reforms in, 178–179
    inconsistency in, 33–35
    loopholes in, 36–37
    Massachusetts 1785 legislation and, 34, 35f
    outside US, 49
    recalls and, 43–48
    testing and, 39–43
    weakened, 115
religion
    bottled water restrictions and, 138–141
    Holy Drinking Water and, 136–137
    holy waters and, 136–138, 139f
    Kabbalah and, 132–135
    unholy purposes and, 132
    water's role in, 131
repackaged recycling, 99
restaurants, 10, 152–154
revolts
    by cities, 147–152
    civil movement and, 158–159
    countering, 159–161
    examples of, 146–147
    Google and, 143
    Idyllwild and, 154–155
    Los Angeles'/Salt Lake City's, 149
    media reports and, 143–144

Nestlé and, 156–157
New York's, 148
other cities', 150
Paris', 147–148
restaurants and, 152–154
sales drop and, 145–146
Seattle's, 150
at source, 154–157
state's, 150
taxes and, 151
tight budgets and, 148, 150
water fountains and, 151–152
Rhythm Structured H2O™, 125
Rochdale, England, 149
Roman water fountains, 18
Rybak, R.T., 149

Safe Drinking Water Act (SDWA), 29,
    185n13
safety, plastic bottle, 90–91
Salazar, Fernando, 10
Salt Lake City, 149
San Leandro plant, 79–80
Sanctuary Springs, Michigan, 75
Schneider, Andrew, 98
Schochet, Immanuel, 132
Schultz, Howard, 167
SDWA. See Safe Drinking Water Act
Seattle, 150
Second Water Age, x, 172–173, 174
selling bottled water
    clustered water, 123–126
    consumer protection and, 116
    decline in, 145–146
    history surrounding, 110–111
    internet and, 115, 117
    oxygen water, 118–121
    Penta Water, 126–130
    prevalence of false claims in, 117–118
    pseudoscience and, 114–115
    weakened regulation and, 115
    weight-loss scams, 121–123
A Short Course in International Marketing
    Blunders (White), 47
Sirico, Robert, 140–141
slogans, 110
Smith, Fred, 8–9
Smith, Michael, 163

snake-oil, 110–111
Snow, John, 24–25, 24f
soft drinks
    beverage sales and, 12–13, 12f
    competition argument concerning,
        11–12
soft path vision, xi, 174–175, 177–178
sommeliers, 84–85
source
    of Cabazon plant water, 65–66
    clean water, 25–26
    confusion, 54, 56–58, 57t
    Poland Spring, 51, 53
    revolt against bottled water and,
        154–157
    taste impacted by, 82–83
sparkling bottled water, 55, 83
Spears, Britney, 135
Spokojny, Artur, 136
spring water. See also Arrowhead Spring
        Water; Arrowhead Spring Water
        Cabazon plant; ground water; Holy
        Spring Water
    designation of, 72
    municipal water compared with, 76
    pathogenic organisms and, 76–78
    Standards of Identity and, 55
    taste regarding, 83
    types of, 67–68
Standards of Identity, 54, 55
Starbucks, 45, 167
sterile water, 55
sterilization, 27
Stevens, Craig, 96
Stroud, Chuck, 154

tap water
    Brita maligning, 10–11
    CEI project and, 9
    Coca-Cola campaign against, 9–10
    coliform bacteria and, 37–38
    competition argument concerning,
        11–12
    cost of convenience and, 95
    Cryptosporidium in, 76
    current challenges regarding, 30–31
    decrease in consumption of, 12–13, 12f
    fear of, 6–8, 17, 30–31

future reforms for, 178
headlines on, 30–31
IBWA and, 7–8
New York City, 17–18, 25–26, 148
Paris and, 147–148
restaurants and, 10, 152–154
taste tests with, 81
war on, 6–13
taste
advertising/marketing influencing, 82
experts in, 81–82
minerals and, 83–84
natural mineral waters and, 83
nature of, 80
Penn and Teller debunking, 85–86
pixie dust and, 80
sommeliers and, 84–85
source impacting, 82–83
tests, 81
Teller. See Penn and Teller
testing
entities carrying out, 40–41
"excessive" label and, 42
FDA, 40–41, 42–43
GAO report on, 39–43
inadequacies of, 40
politicians on, 43
taste and, 81
Think Outside the Bottle campaign, 158
Third Age of Water
hard path vision of, x–xi, 175–177
soft path vision of, xi, 174–175,
177–178
Thirsty Planet, 168
Thum, Peter, 165–167
transportation, 94–95

UCC. See United Church of Canada
UCF. See University of Central Florida

United Church of Canada (UCC), 139
University of Central Florida (UCF), 1–3

Villaraigosa, Antonio, 149
Vitamin O, 120–121

Wallace, Sir Richard, 19, 147
water fountains
American cities and, 19–21
disappearance of, 3, 106–107
future reforms for, 178
Greeks/Romans and, 18
history regarding, 3–4, 18–21
London and, 18–19
New York City, 20–21
Paris, 19
resurgence of, 151–152
UCF and, 1–3
Waters, Alice, 153
Waxman, Henry A., 42
weight, of water, 88
weight-loss scams
FTC and, 121–122
hydroxycitric acid and, 123
Jana Skinny Water, 122–123
panoply of, 122
well water, 55
Wellington, Susan, 1, 7
Whinfield, John Rex, 87, 88
White, Michael, 47
William, King of England, 21–22
wine taste, 81–82
Wolpe, David, 132

Young, James Harvey, 111

Zephyrhills, 156, 160
Zunami water, 126

About Island Press

Since 1984, the nonprofit Island Press has been stimulating, shaping, and communicating the ideas that are essential for solving environmental problems worldwide. With more than 800 titles in print and some 40 new releases each year, we are the nation's leading publisher on environmental issues. We identify innovative thinkers and emerging trends in the environmental field. We work with world-renowned experts and authors to develop cross-disciplinary solutions to environmental challenges.

Island Press designs and implements coordinated book publication campaigns in order to communicate our critical messages in print, in person, and online using the latest technologies, programs, and the media. Our goal: to reach targeted audiences—scientists, policymakers, environmental advocates, the media, and concerned citizens—who can and will take action to protect the plants and animals that enrich our world, the ecosystems we need to survive, the water we drink, and the air we breathe.

Island Press gratefully acknowledges the support of its work by the Agua Fund, Inc., The Margaret A. Cargill Foundation, Betsy and Jesse Fink Foundation, The William and Flora Hewlett Foundation, The Kresge Foundation, The Forrest and Frances Lattner Foundation, The Andrew W. Mellon Foundation, The Curtis and Edith Munson Foundation, The Overbrook Foundation, The David and Lucile Packard Foundation, The Summit Foundation, Trust for Architectural Easements, The Winslow Foundation, and other generous donors.

The opinions expressed in this book are those of the author(s) and do not necessarily reflect the views of our donors.